Getting into University

Veterinary School

Emily Lucas

14th edition

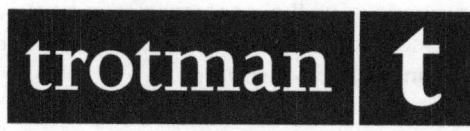

Getting into University: Veterinary School

This 14th edition published in 2026 by Trotman, an imprint of Trotman Indigo Publishing Ltd, 18e Charles Street, Bath BA1 1HX

© Trotman Indigo Publishing Ltd 2026

Author: Emily Lucas
12th–13th edn: Emily Lucas
7th–11th edns: James Barton
5th–6th edns: Mario De Clemente
3rd–4th edns: James Burnett
1st–2nd edns: John Handley (published as Getting into Veterinary Science)

Editions 1–6 published by Trotman and Co. Ltd

British Library Cataloguing in Publication Data
A catalogue record for this book is available from the British Library.

Paperback ISBN 978 1 911724 97 1
eISBN 978 1 911724 98 8

All rights reserved. This book is sold subject to the condition that it shall not, by way of trade or otherwise, be lent, resold, hired out or otherwise circulated without the publisher's prior written consent in any form of binding or cover other than that in which it is published and without a similar condition including this condition being imposed on the subsequent purchaser. No part of this publication may be reproduced, stored in a retrieval system or transmitted in any form or by any means, electronic and mechanical, photocopying, recording or otherwise without prior permission of Trotman Indigo Publishing.

Every effort has been made to trace copyright holders and to obtain their permission for the use of copyright material. The publisher apologises for any errors or omissions, and would be grateful to be notified of any corrections that should be incorporated in future editions of this book.

The authorised representative in the EEA is Easy Access System Europe Oü (EAS), Mustamäe tee 50, 10621 Tallinn, Estonia.

Printed and bound in the UK by 4edge Ltd, Hockley, Essex.

 All details in this book were correct at the time of going to press. To keep up to date with all the latest news and updates and to access the online resources that accompany this book, use this QR code or visit **www.trotman.co.uk/pages/getting-into-online-resources**.

Contents

	About the author	vi
	Acknowledgements	vii
	Introduction: 'Do I have a cat in hell's chance?!'	1
	Veterinary medicine as a profession	1
	What veterinary schools look for	2
	Using this book	2
1|	**The bare necessities: What is the role of a vet?**	**7**
	Beyond treatment: education and prevention	7
	Continuous professional development	8
	The modern veterinary role	8
	What makes a good vet?	8
	Prevention	9
	Small animal practice	10
	Large animal practice	11
	So why do you want to be a vet?	11
2|	**Horses for courses: Studying veterinary medicine**	**15**
	Accreditation and course structure	15
	From foundations to practice	16
	Different schools, different styles	16
	The bigger picture	16
	The pre-clinical stage (Years 1–2)	17
	The para-clinical stage (Years 2–3)	18
	The clinical stage (Years 4–5)	19
	Extramural studies (EMS)	20
	Veterinary course types and entry routes	21
	Notes on veterinary courses in the UK	23
3|	**Separating the sheep from the goats: Preparation and experience**	**29**
	Starting early	29
	Getting more experience	30
	Specific university requirements	31
	Making the initial contact	33
	What to expect from a veterinary placement	34
	Making a positive impression in practice	34
	Variety and commitment	37
	Getting the most out of your work experience	38
	Online work experience	40
	Beyond work experience	40

4| The 'Jack Russell' group: Choosing your course — 43
- Choice of school — 43
- Course entry requirements — 45
- Academic and subject requirements — 46
- Choosing your A levels — 46
- Other qualifications — 51
- Choosing the right veterinary school: a checklist — 53
- The fifth choice — 54

5| Take the bull by the horns in the cattle market: The UCAS application — 57
- What happens to your application? — 58
- Submitting your application — 61
- The reference — 62
- What happens next? — 63
- Other supporting documentation — 65
- Admissions tests — 66
- UCAS Extra — 66
- What to do if you are rejected — 67
- Deferring entry and taking a gap year — 68
- Transferring from another degree — 68

6| No one likes a copycat: The personal statement — 73
- What admissions tutors are looking for — 73
- Sections of the personal statement — 74
- Summary: planning your responses — 76
- Using Artificial Intelligence (AI) in your UCAS application — 77
- Things to avoid — 78
- Example personal statements — 80
- General tips — 86

7| So why did the chicken cross the road?: The interview — 87
- The purpose of the interview — 87
- Preparing for your veterinary school interview — 89
- How to succeed in the interview — 92
- General interview tips — 95
- How you are selected — 96
- What happens next? — 97
- Topical and controversial issues — 98
- Breeding, science and ethics — 107
- Other issues — 110
- Topical issues summary — 113
- Importance of the interview — 115

8| A leopard does not change its spots: Non-standard applicants — 117
- International and EU applicants — 117
- Studying outside the UK — 119
- Mature students — 120

Students with disabilities and additional learning needs	120
Gateway and Foundation programmes	121
Graduate entry into veterinary medicine	122

9| A bird in the hand: Results day — 125

When the results are available	125
What to do if you have no offers: UCAS Extra	125
What to do if things go wrong during the exams	126
What to do on results day	126
What to do if you exceeded the grades that you expected	127
What to do if you have no confirmed offers	128
UCAS Clearing	128
If you decide to retake your A levels	129
If you decide to reapply	130

10| Counting sheep: Financing your course — 131

Fees	132
Living expenses	133
Funding	134
Keeping costs down: hints and tips	138

11| Snakes and ladders: Career paths — 141

Veterinary Graduate Development Programme (VetGDP)	141
Career opportunities	142
Postgraduate courses	143
Veterinary variety: types of vet	144
The veterinary practice	149
Accreditation	151
Government and military service	152
Veterinary teaching and research	153
Charity and welfare organisations	154
Non-clinical veterinary careers	155
Veterinary salaries and career progression	157
Veterinary nurses	159
Women in the profession	161
Wellbeing in the veterinary profession	161
Summing up	163
The unique skills a vet requires	164

12| Don't count your chickens before they've hatched: Further information — 165

Veterinary schools in the UK	165
Other contacts and sources of information	168

Glossary — 171

About the author

Emily Lucas read medical science at the University of Birmingham before obtaining a master's degree in genomic medicine from Queen Mary, University of London. She currently holds the position of University Support Officer at MPW, and helps students with their university applications, as well as supporting students with pre-admissions tests. As well as teaching biology, Emily is currently undertaking a PhD in neuroscience at the University of Southampton. She is the current co-author of Trotman's *Getting into University: Dental School* and *Medical School* guides.

Acknowledgements

I would like to thank everybody who has contributed to the thirteenth edition of *Getting into University: Veterinary School*, including MPW and Trotman for giving me the opportunity to write it.

I would like to thank all of the individuals who have contributed to the book, especially Amira D, Marie K, Bex W, Melisa K, Sophie J, Sophie L, Hannah S, James H and Georgia O for their insights into applying to, studying and working in the field of veterinary medicine. In addition, I would like to thank James H, Georgia O, Maria L and former contributors for allowing me to reproduce their personal statements here as successful examples. I am extremely grateful that these individuals were willing to take time out of their busy schedules to contribute.

I would also like to thank those at UCAS and the Royal College of Veterinary Surgeons, as well as the university admissions departments, who have supported me by answering questions and providing statistics.

Emily Lucas

Introduction
'Do I have a cat in hell's chance?!'

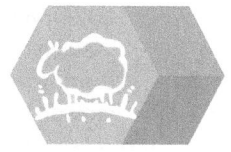

Applying to veterinary school is both exciting and demanding. It requires careful preparation, thoughtful reflection and a genuine understanding of what a career in veterinary medicine involves. This book will guide you through each stage of the process, from exploring your motivation and gaining the right experience to preparing your personal statement and interviews, helping you to present yourself as a well-informed and committed applicant.

Success rarely comes overnight. The most competitive applicants start planning early, researching courses thoroughly and building relevant experience over time. A steady, organised approach will always put you in a stronger position than a last-minute rush.

The process of applying to veterinary school can be challenging, but it is also a valuable opportunity for growth. Each step allows you to deepen your understanding of the profession, strengthen your communication skills and demonstrate your commitment to animal welfare and science.

By the end of this book, you will have a clear picture of what veterinary schools are looking for and how to stand out from the crowd. With preparation, persistence and genuine enthusiasm, you'll be ready to take the next step towards joining one of the most respected and rewarding professions – proof, perhaps, that every dog really does have its day.

Veterinary medicine as a profession

Veterinary medicine is far more than a career for animal lovers – it's a vital profession that protects animal health, supports public wellbeing and safeguards the environment. Vets are central to the One Health movement, which recognises the close connection between human, animal and ecosystem health. Whether treating companion animals, supporting livestock and food production, conducting biomedical research or advising on policy and biosecurity, vets play a crucial role in improving lives on a global scale.

The landscape of veterinary education and practice continues to evolve. New veterinary schools, such as those at Harper & Keele (fully accredited in 2024) and the University of Lancashire (launched in 2024), have expanded opportunities for applicants, while advances in medical technology, genetics and animal welfare science are reshaping the profession. Increasing awareness of sustainability, antibiotic stewardship and animal ethics means that future vets must be not only scientifically skilled but also adaptable, reflective and ethically aware.

What veterinary schools look for

Academic excellence will always be essential, particularly in the sciences, but veterinary schools are also looking for empathy, resilience and strong communication skills. Vets work closely with owners, farmers and colleagues, often in emotionally charged situations. Understanding the human side of veterinary medicine – being able to listen, explain and reassure – is as important as technical ability.

The competition is fierce, and not every applicant will be successful the first time, but persistence and self-awareness go a long way. Many vets reach their goal through alternative routes, reapplication or postgraduate entry. Each stage of the process, from work experience to interview, helps you grow in confidence, reflection and understanding of what it truly means to join this profession.

Using this book

Applying to veterinary school is an exciting but demanding process. Each year, thousands of applicants compete for a limited number of places, and success depends on strong preparation, academic ability and a genuine understanding of what life as a vet involves.

According to the UCAS End-of-Cycle 2024 data, there were 11,705 applications for veterinary medicine and dentistry in the UK, with 3,580 offers made – an offer rate of around 30%. Of those, only about 1,200 students went on to take up places on accredited veterinary programmes leading to registration with the Royal College of Veterinary Surgeons (RCVS).

This book is your step-by-step guide to navigating that journey. It will help you to research veterinary courses, plan your application, gain relevant work experience, write your personal statement and prepare for interview. You'll also find advice for mature applicants, graduates and international students, along with sections on student finance, results day and career options after qualification.

Each chapter tackles a different stage of the process, using examples, student insights and practical advice to help you prepare effectively:

1. **The bare necessities**: what is the role of a vet?
2. **Horses for courses**: studying veterinary medicine.
3. **Separating the sheep from the goats**: preparation and experience.
4. **The 'Jack Russell' group**: choosing your course.
5. **Take the bull by the horns**: completing the UCAS application.
6. **No one likes a copycat**: writing your personal statement.
7. **So why did the chicken cross the road?**: the interview.
8. **A leopard does not change its spots**: non-standard applicants.
9. **A bird in the hand**: results day and reapplications.
10. **Counting sheep**: financing your course.
11. **Snakes and ladders**: veterinary careers and specialisms.
12. **Don't count your chickens before they've hatched**: further resources and glossary.

While this book focuses on the application process, it will also help you decide whether veterinary medicine is truly the right career for you. Academic ability, particularly in science, is essential, but so too are communication, empathy and resilience. Every animal you treat will bring a human story with it, and how you handle both will define you as a vet.

Throughout the book, you'll find real student insights, offering first-hand advice from those who've been through the process. Their experiences will help you to understand both the challenges and rewards of training as a vet and to approach your own application with confidence and clarity.

Case study

Melisa is a final year student at the Royal Veterinary College (RVC).

'Having now finished all of my training, lectures and rotations at RVC, I am now just preparing for my final year exams before graduating and being able to practise as a veterinarian.

'I eventually want to have my own vet clinic, where I hope to predominantly take care of small pets and exotic species. Before that though, I am hoping to secure a job in a clinic in order to gain more first-hand experience of what this role entails on a full-time basis and, more importantly, get a better understanding of the management side of the role.

'It was my love of animals that motivated me to want to be a vet, and especially wanting to care for them. As I grew older, I realised it would be a real privilege to be able to turn this passion into my job, and I am genuinely excited to be able to wake up every day and do what I love for the rest of my life, and earn a living doing it. It was this that pushed me through the tough years of revision and exams as I worked towards getting a place on a veterinary medicine degree and then succeeding in it.

'Perhaps an area that I appreciated less when applying was how important it is to build relationships with the owners of the animals, rather than just working with the animals themselves. Through extensive placements in hospitals and clinics, I have learned to really enjoy this element of the role. It is very rewarding to be able to help owners' pets return to full health, and to be there for the owners when things get challenging.

'The diagnostics element of the job is something that I find very stimulating, as you have to hone in on clues about the case presented by the owner, given that you can't get information from the patient themselves. When tied in with the psychology of dealing with emotional owners, it is a very rounded and rewarding job. The added bonus is being able to deal with so many animals, many of which are species I wouldn't encounter on a daily basis!

'Though the end of my degree is in sight now, with just my final exams to go, the hardest part of the degree for me was the countless days and nights of revision. However, I found ways to make revision more fun and strategies that have got me through the last five years.

'I also initially had a hard time adjusting to the fact that it is okay to not always know the right answer, and that even the best vets in the world aren't always able to come up with a diagnosis; the important thing is to be able to help these animals in the best way that we can, given the circumstances.

'There are some interesting areas in veterinary medicine at the moment, including animal products production, and the effects of this on the environment as well as human health and safety, such as zoonotic diseases and food safety. Another hot topic is vaccines – a shortage of veterinary vaccines still continues post-Covid, which leads to many pets not being able to get vaccinated and catching diseases that are lethal but normally preventable. Linked to this is traceability and surveillance of diseases in animals. TB (tuberculosis) continues to be a persistent problem, but more recently, rabies has emerged as an issue due to puppies having fake vaccination statuses.

'To any aspiring vets, I would say that when things get hard, you always need to remember why you first started chasing your dreams, and use that to keep pushing through to the light at the end of the tunnel.

'In terms of advice for the application, I would recommend getting as much work experience as possible in different fields. Rather than doing a bunch of weeks in just a regular clinic, try to include other areas, such as husbandry experiences in stud farms, lambing experiences, overseas pre-vet volunteering programmes and animal shelters. I found that this was definitely one of the most important things to be able to show and talk about at interview, as admissions officers expect you to be fully aware of the broad spectrum of learning you will have to do. As I had a lot of experiences in different fields, I was actually made an offer with a lower grade than my colleagues that year.

'In preparation for interviews, have a look at general medical interview questions, and be prepared to answer questions such as why you want to work with animals rather than humans (bearing in mind they are trying to make sure that you understand every animal comes with an owner, possibly even two, so if you don't like dealing with people, this will be a red flag in the interview). They also like you to demonstrate how you would cope with stressful conversations with owners, so it is important to go over communication skills and techniques. They also like to check candidates' manual dexterity and instruction-following skills, typically by asking you to follow basic instructions to build something. Finally, one of the most important things in the interview is to be respectful yet sure of yourself and your abilities – be outgoing about these as they want to see your true personality and how you can advocate for yourself in different situations.'

Fact: Almost half the pigs in the world are kept by farmers in China.

1 | The bare necessities
What is the role of a vet?

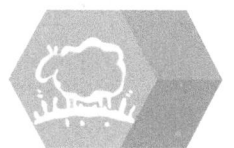

This is perhaps the most fundamental question of all, because the answer reflects the considerable commitment, of time, energy and empathy, that every vet makes. Veterinary practice is not a nine-to-five career. Under the RCVS Code of Professional Conduct, veterinary surgeons must take steps to ensure 24-hour access to emergency first aid and pain relief, whether delivered by the practice itself or via an appropriate out-of-hours provider. As one farmer put it, a vet needs a good sense of humour to be called out at 3 a.m. on a freezing night to deliver a calf, knee-deep in mud.

It is certainly not a profession for the hesitant or uncertain. Vets are held in high esteem, viewed as skilled, compassionate and dedicated professionals who put animal welfare first. The best vets combine scientific expertise with calm decision-making, communication skills and genuine care – qualities that underpin every successful practice.

The enduring popularity of James Herriot's stories reflects how the public values the profession: real triumphs and challenges, constant learning and a genuine love of the work.

Beyond treatment: education and prevention

The role of the vet is about much more than clinical expertise. Education and prevention are central to the profession. Vets advise owners, farmers and the wider public on animal health and welfare, helping to prevent disease and promote responsible care.

In large animal practice, this might mean advising on herd management to reduce infection risk. In small animal practice, it could involve helping new pet owners understand vaccination, nutrition or behavioural needs. In every case, effective communication is essential – translating complex science into practical advice that protects both animal and human wellbeing.

Continuous professional development

Veterinary medicine is constantly evolving, and lifelong learning is a professional obligation. Veterinary surgeons must complete a minimum of 35 hours of CPD each year (veterinary nurses 15 hours), recorded in the RCVS 1CPD platform with reflective practice to help link learning to real-world cases. Activities range from clinical-skills workshops and research projects to in-house training and 'seeing practice'.

Examples of CPD include:

- clinical-skills workshops or practical training;
- discussion groups or learning sets;
- preparing lectures or presentations;
- research or audit projects;
- secondments or work-based observation ('seeing practice');
- in-house or external training courses.

The modern veterinary role

Today's vets work in an extraordinary range of settings, from companion animal practice to wildlife conservation, research, government service and the pharmaceutical industry. The modern vet is not only a clinician but also a communicator, scientist, educator and advocate for animal welfare.

They contribute to the global One Health agenda, recognising the interconnectedness of animal, human and environmental health. Preventative care also supports national efforts on antimicrobial stewardship, helping to tackle resistance across both animal and human medicine. Vets play key roles in food safety, disease control and sustainability, and increasingly they champion mental health awareness within the profession itself, through initiatives such as the RCVS Mind Matters Initiative.

New UK graduates also complete the Veterinary Graduate Development Programme (VetGDP), a structured period of mentored practice that replaced the Professional Development Phase (PDP) in 2021, supporting the transition from student to practising vet.

What makes a good vet?

Veterinary medicine demands a unique combination of personal and professional qualities. Vets must be scientists, problem solvers, communicators and decision-makers – often all within the same consultation. No two days are ever the same, and the ability to stay calm, confident and compassionate under pressure is key.

1 | What Is the Role of a Vet?

A good vet demonstrates:

- **Confidence and composure**: staying calm under pressure and communicating decisions clearly.
- **Authority and professionalism**: inspiring trust from clients and colleagues alike.
- **Empathy**: showing genuine care for both animals and their owners;
- **Resilience**: coping with long hours, emotional challenges and unpredictable cases.
- **Focus and organisation:** balancing multiple responsibilities without losing attention to detail.
- **Good judgement**: weighing prevention against treatment, and science against practicality.
- **Versatility**: adapting to new technologies, species and clinical settings.
- **Self-awareness**: recognising when to seek advice or refer a case.
- **Lifelong learning**: staying informed about advances in medicine, welfare and ethics.

Veterinary work can be demanding, and resilience is an essential part of success. Vets face physical and emotional challenges daily, from handling emergencies and making difficult decisions to supporting clients through the loss of an animal. The ability to remain composed and compassionate, even in difficult moments, defines the best practitioners.

Newly qualified vets, in particular, need to balance confidence with humility. It takes maturity to recognise when you need help or a second opinion, and that awareness is a mark of professionalism, not weakness. The veterinary profession thrives on collaboration, mentorship and continual learning. Knowing your limits and seeking guidance when needed is part of being a responsible and effective vet.

Prevention

Even with the technological advances of the 21st century, the principle remains the same: prevention is better than cure. Animals cannot explain when they are unwell, so one of a vet's most important responsibilities is to anticipate and prevent disease wherever possible.

Preventative veterinary medicine covers everything from vaccination schedules and parasite control to biosecurity, nutrition and welfare management. Good vets think ahead, advising clients when and how to protect their animals, rather than waiting until illness occurs. For example, suggesting the right time for herd vaccination before winter respiratory disease, or improving housing to prevent lameness, demonstrates both foresight and professionalism.

Preventative care benefits everyone: it improves animal welfare, supports productivity and reduces the need for antibiotics, helping to combat antimicrobial resistance and supporting the wider One Health agenda. It also strengthens the trust between vet and client, as proactive advice often prevents costly emergencies later on.

However, prevention is not always straightforward. It can be expensive, and in agriculture especially, financial pressures may lead farmers to delay veterinary visits until problems arise. The role of the vet is therefore as much about education and diplomacy as it is about medicine – explaining the long-term benefits of good husbandry and helping clients make informed, sustainable choices.

Sometimes, the most valuable advice a vet gives is simple but practical: improving housing, adjusting feed composition or altering a routine that causes unnecessary stress or injury. The best vets combine scientific knowledge with keen observation and common sense, using evidence-based prevention to promote both welfare and productivity.

Small animal practice

Working with household pets requires a different set of skills from large animal or farm work. It is as much about supporting and counselling the owners as it is about treating the patients themselves, and strong interpersonal skills are essential.

Small animal practice offers extraordinary variety. In a single day, a vet might diagnose a nutritional problem in a reptile, investigate weight loss in a cat, treat a rabbit for myxomatosis or simply microchip a new puppy for security. Dental disease, obesity and age-related conditions are common challenges, and vets must often balance medical expertise with persuasive communication, encouraging owners to make sustainable changes in diet, exercise or lifestyle for the benefit of their pets.

Many small animal vets work in busy urban practices, where road traffic accidents and emergency cases are frequent. In critical situations, a calm and organised approach can mean the difference between life and death. Every second counts, but the true professional remains composed, prepared and decisive under pressure.

Perhaps the most emotionally demanding part of small animal practice is making decisions about euthanasia. While the ethical questions differ from those in human medicine, the emotional weight can be just as heavy. Vets must balance the animal's welfare, the owner's wishes and their own professional judgement when deciding whether euthanasia is the kindest option.

Empathy and communication are vital. Owners often see their pets as members of the family, and breaking difficult news requires compassion, sensitivity and clarity. The way a vet supports an owner through loss can have a lasting impact, not only on that relationship but on the owner's future willingness to seek veterinary care.

For many vets, euthanasia remains one of the hardest aspects of the job, despite being an act of kindness. Handling these moments with dignity and understanding is one of the clearest demonstrations of what it means to be a veterinary professional.

Large animal practice

Caring for large animals requires a distinct skill set and mindset. The work is physically demanding and often unpredictable, and it calls for confidence, calmness and quick decision-making. Large animals are powerful and sensitive to body language; a vet who is hesitant or unsure may find them difficult to handle. Gaining an animal's trust requires assurance and composure as well as technical skill.

Farmers form quick judgements based on how a vet handles livestock. A calm, efficient and proactive manner builds trust, while hesitation can undermine it. Clear communication, teamwork and respect for the farmer's expertise sustain long-term relationships and better herd outcomes.

Working with farmers also demands diplomacy and understanding. For many farmers, animals are both a livelihood and a source of personal pride. Vets must respect this dual perspective – recognising that decisions about herd health, culling or treatment affect not only welfare but also business viability. Communicating clearly and empathetically, while maintaining professional authority, is key to building lasting trust.

Large animal vets must also approach their patients differently from small animal clinicians. Their focus is on herd and population health as much as on individual cases. The work combines preventative care, disease control and welfare management, from fertility checks and calving to nutrition and vaccination programmes. Many of these animals are raised for food or work, and vets must be able to separate personal emotion from professional responsibility while still advocating for humane and ethical treatment.

So why do you want to be a vet?

It's one of the most important questions you can ask yourself, and one that admissions tutors will ask too. Becoming a vet means choosing a career that is demanding, rewarding and often all-consuming. For many people, it's more than a job; it's a way of life.

A love of animals is, of course, expected, but it isn't enough on its own. What truly defines a good vet is how you respond when faced with challenge or uncertainty. Emergencies rarely happen at convenient times, and success often depends on your ability to stay calm, think clearly and act decisively. The satisfaction comes not from recognition, but from knowing you have made a difference, whether by saving a life, easing pain or helping an owner understand what their animal needs.

Commitment is essential. Veterinary medicine requires long hours of study, resilience through setbacks, and the determination to keep learning throughout your career. For most vets, that commitment begins early and deepens with experience – through volunteering, work placements and the growing realisation that this is not just something they enjoy, but something they need to do.

While many qualified vets work in clinical practice, this is only one of many possible paths. Some go on to specialise in surgery, research or pathology; others pursue careers in teaching, public health, animal welfare or government inspection. Whatever direction you take, the same principles apply: curiosity, compassion and the commitment to use your knowledge for the benefit of animals, people and society as a whole.

Case study

Sophie studied A levels in biology, chemistry and psychology, achieving A*AA and securing a place on the BVSc Veterinary Science degree at the University of Bristol.

Sophie's story highlights the importance of early preparation, reflection and resilience. Veterinary medicine is an intellectually demanding and emotionally challenging degree, but students who plan ahead, balance their wellbeing and approach each experience with curiosity and openness are well placed to thrive.

'I always knew I wanted a career that combined science and helping animals, but I didn't fully understand what being a vet involved until I started work experience. I spent time at a small animal practice, a dairy farm and a wildlife rescue centre. Each setting gave me a completely different view of the profession, from the practical side of farm visits to the emotional side of working with pets and their owners. That variety really confirmed this was what I wanted to do.

'Every university seems to ask for something slightly different, so I started researching requirements in Year 12 and logged everything I did. I ended up with around ten weeks' experience split between small animal, equine and farm work. It's not about ticking boxes – it's about understanding what daily life as a vet is really like.

'A levels were intense, especially while trying to fit in early mornings on farms, but the experience gave me a good work ethic. The main thing universities look for is reflection; they want to see that you've learned from each placement, not just that you've been there.

'Vet school is rewarding but demanding. The workload can be heavy and you don't get as much time off as other students because placements take up most of your holidays. At times it can feel overwhelming, but I've learned to set boundaries and prioritise rest. The staff are supportive, and there's a real sense of community within the vet school as everyone looks out for each other.

'When I started, I only imagined myself in small animal practice, but through lectures and EMS placements, I've become really interested in public health and disease control. I like the idea of working in an area that links animal and human health, maybe with the APHA or in a research setting. There are so many career paths you don't realise exist when you first apply.

'Start early with your work experience and keep a reflective diary. It makes your personal statement much stronger. Don't worry if you don't have it all figured out – most students change their mind about what kind of vet they want to be several times during the course. And take care of yourself. Vet school can be intense, but it's also an incredible opportunity to learn, grow and find where you fit in the profession.'

Fact: Cows form best friends, and get stressed when they're separated.

2 | Horses for courses
Studying veterinary medicine

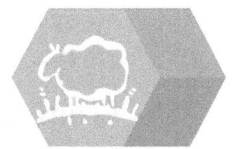

Applying to veterinary school is one of the most competitive academic challenges in the UK, so it can feel unusual to think of having a choice of courses. Yet each year, many successful applicants find themselves holding two or more offers and facing the question: which vet school is right for me?

Often, this decision is made on personal factors – the feel of the campus at an open day, recommendations from current students or proximity to home. While these are perfectly valid, it's also worth understanding how veterinary degrees differ in structure, emphasis and teaching style. A little research now will help you make a more confident and informed decision later, and may even give you useful examples to discuss in interviews.

Accreditation and course structure

All UK veterinary degrees must meet the requirements of the Royal College of Veterinary Surgeons (RCVS) under the Veterinary Surgeons Act 1966. Only graduates from RCVS-accredited programmes are eligible to join the RCVS Register of Veterinary Surgeons, which confers the legal right to practise as a vet in the UK.

This means that, although the UK's veterinary schools vary in teaching style and emphasis, they share a common core of professional outcomes. Each school must ensure that students graduate with the 'Day One Competences' defined by the RCVS – the essential knowledge, skills and professional attributes required for safe, independent practice.

Because of these shared standards, the overall structure of each degree is broadly similar, even if the detail differs from one school to another. All programmes integrate pre-clinical, para-clinical and clinical phases, moving gradually from foundational science to hands-on practice. In most cases, this takes five years, although accelerated graduate-entry routes and six-year widening participation pathways are available at some universities.

From foundations to practice

The early years of the degree focus on the basic and biomedical sciences that underpin animal health and disease. You'll study subjects such as anatomy, physiology, biochemistry, genetics, pharmacology and animal husbandry, often using a combination of lectures, dissections, lab practicals and problem-based learning.

As you progress, these topics are applied to real-world scenarios in the para-clinical and clinical years. You'll learn how diseases develop, how they are diagnosed and treated and how different body systems interact. This stage is when the theory starts to make sense: everything from molecular biology to animal handling begins to connect to the realities of patient care.

In the later years, students spend increasing time in clinical rotations and extramural studies (EMS), gaining direct experience in small animal, equine, farm and public health settings. These placements allow you to apply your knowledge, develop professional confidence and experience the wide variety of roles a vet can take on.

Different schools, different styles

Although all UK vet schools lead to the same professional qualification, they vary in size, facilities and teaching methods. Some, like Cambridge and Edinburgh, follow a more traditional science-led model with a strong research base. Others, such as Nottingham and Surrey, emphasise integrated or problem-based learning, where scientific knowledge and clinical reasoning are taught together from the start.

Newer schools, including Harper & Keele and the University of Lancashire, have introduced modern facilities and smaller cohort sizes, focusing on community practice and employability. Each school has its own culture, so visiting open days, speaking to current students and reading RCVS accreditation reports can help you decide which environment suits your learning style best.

The bigger picture

While the science is challenging, veterinary education is designed to produce reflective, adaptable professionals. You will be expected not only to master technical knowledge but also to communicate effectively, make ethical decisions and work safely as part of a multidisciplinary team.

The course is long and demanding, but it offers unparalleled variety. One week you might be learning about the genetics of disease, and the next you could be assisting in surgery, monitoring anaesthesia or working on herd health management during an EMS placement.

Whatever vet school you choose, your journey will combine academic study, professional growth and personal discovery – the very reasons this career remains one of the most respected in the world.

The pre-clinical stage (Years 1–2)

The pre-clinical years focus on the healthy animal. You'll build the scientific foundations that underpin all later clinical work: how bodies are put together, how they function and how animals are cared for. Teaching typically blends lectures, small-group tutorials, lab practicals, dissection/prosection, digital microscopy and early clinical-skills sessions. The goal is simple: understand normal so you can recognise abnormal.

Veterinary anatomy

You'll study structure from cell to system across species, linking gross anatomy (locomotion, musculoskeletal, respiratory, cardiovascular, gastrointestinal, urogenital, nervous systems) with microscopic anatomy (histology). Expect hands-on sessions using models, specimens, imaging and clinical correlations so form is always tied to function (e.g. why equine limb anatomy predisposes to specific injuries).

Physiology and biochemistry

Here you learn how the body works and how systems interact. Core themes include cellular metabolism and homeostasis, neurophysiology, endocrine control, renal and fluid balance, cardiovascular and respiratory physiology, gastrointestinal function and reproduction. You'll apply biochemistry to real veterinary contexts (from energy balance and lactation to pharmacology basics), building the platform for pathophysiology and therapeutics later on.

Genetics, behaviour and animal husbandry

Most programmes integrate genetics and genomics, animal behaviour and welfare and animal husbandry. You'll cover breeding strategies, population traits, preventative health, biosecurity, housing, nutrition and species-specific handling across companion, equine and production animals. Early handling and restraint teaching emphasises safety, welfare and low-stress techniques.

Skills you start building

- **Practical skills**: safe handling and basic procedures, clinical communication, record-keeping and reflection.
- **Scientific skills**: data interpretation, evidence appraisal and fundamental lab techniques.
- **Professional skills**: teamwork, ethics and welfare-first decision-making.

How it joins up later

Content is usually delivered in an integrated or spiral curriculum: you'll revisit systems with increasing clinical depth. What you learn here directly feeds the para-clinical phase (pathology, microbiology/parasitology, immunology, pharmacology) and then your clinical rotations and EMS placements.

The para-clinical stage (Years 2-3)

The para-clinical stage bridges the gap between studying healthy animals and diagnosing disease. You'll apply your scientific foundation to understanding how and why illness occurs, and how it can be prevented or treated. This stage introduces the major disciplines that explain the mechanisms of disease and the principles of therapy.

Pathology

Pathology is the scientific study of disease – what causes it, how it develops and how it affects the body. You'll examine the structural and functional changes that occur in cells, tissues and organs when disease is present, linking what you see under the microscope with what you observe in the clinic. Areas include gross pathology, histopathology, clinical pathology and necropsy techniques. By the end of this phase, you'll understand the patterns of disease across species and the laboratory methods used to confirm a diagnosis.

Microbiology, parasitology and immunology

These subjects explore the infectious agents that cause disease and the body's defences against them. You'll study bacteria, viruses, fungi, protozoa and helminths of veterinary importance, learning how they spread, how to identify them and how to control or eradicate them. Immunology introduces the immune system's role in protection, vaccination, allergy and immune-mediated disease, linking directly to both preventative medicine and public health work.

Pharmacology and therapeutics

Pharmacology focuses on how drugs act, how the body handles them and how to use them safely and effectively. You'll learn about:

- **Pharmacodynamics**: how drugs exert their effects at the molecular and cellular level.
- **Pharmacokinetics**: how drugs are absorbed, distributed, metabolised and excreted.
- **Therapeutics**: how medicines are used to prevent and treat disease across species.

This knowledge underpins rational prescribing, anaesthesia and pain management in the clinical years. Many schools also integrate teaching on antimicrobial stewardship, drug legislation and evidence-based prescribing to prepare you for professional practice.

The clinical stage (Years 4–5)

The clinical stage is where everything you've learnt finally comes together. These final years build on the scientific foundations of the pre-clinical and para-clinical phases, developing your ability to diagnose, treat and prevent disease across a wide range of species. You'll move from classroom-based study to hands-on practice in real clinical settings, gaining the confidence and professional judgement required for independent practice.

Teaching is delivered in small-group rotations, both within university hospitals (intramural rotations) and through external veterinary placements (EMS). You'll work alongside clinicians in areas such as medicine, surgery, anaesthesia, reproduction, diagnostic imaging and population health.

Many schools also introduce public health and food safety, preparing you for roles that extend beyond companion and farm animals, from meat hygiene and zoonotic disease control to One Health and biosecurity.

Clinical learning and practical skills

You'll develop a wide range of practical and professional competences, guided by the RCVS Day One Competences, which define the skills every graduate must have before entering practice. This includes:

- clinical examination and diagnostic techniques (from imaging and laboratory testing to ultrasound and endoscopy);
- safe administration of anaesthesia and analgesia;
- surgical principles, asepsis and wound management;
- reproductive medicine, including obstetrics and neonatal care;

- herd and flock health, preventative medicine and client communication;
- record-keeping, ethics and welfare-first decision-making.

You'll also refine your soft skills, including leadership, teamwork, communication and reflection, which are just as vital as technical ability.

From student to professional

As you rotate through small animal, equine and farm animal practice, you'll begin to see how theory translates into clinical reasoning. Each case will draw on your earlier learning in anatomy, physiology, pathology and pharmacology. It's often during these years that students say everything finally clicks and they start to think and act like vets.

Clinical placements can be demanding. You may face long days, early mornings and on-call work, sometimes in less-than-ideal weather conditions. But this is also the most rewarding part of the degree – the moment when your skills, confidence and compassion converge. You'll graduate with the knowledge, competence and professional insight needed to begin your first role as a qualified veterinary surgeon.

Extramural studies (EMS)

Extramural studies (EMS) form a core part of every UK veterinary degree. They provide essential, hands-on experience outside the university setting and are designed to complement your formal teaching. EMS placements give you the chance to apply what you've learnt, gain confidence handling animals and develop practical skills in real-world environments.

Two types of EMS

The Royal College of Veterinary Surgeons (RCVS) requires all students to complete a minimum of 38 weeks of approved EMS before graduation, divided into two stages:

- **Animal Husbandry EMS (AHEMS)**: usually 12 weeks during the first two years of study. This stage focuses on understanding how animals are reared, handled and cared for. Students typically work on farms, in kennels, catteries, stables or other animal facilities to develop safe handling techniques and an appreciation of animal welfare and production systems.
- **Clinical EMS (CEMS)**: usually 26 weeks spread across the later years of the course. This involves supervised placements in veterinary practices and related organisations, including small animal, equine, farm animal, mixed or specialist settings. Students may also spend shorter periods in laboratories, diagnostic centres,

abattoirs or public health environments to gain broader professional experience.

Organisation and support

Students are responsible for arranging their own EMS placements, though every veterinary school provides approved provider lists, placement databases and support teams to help with organisation. The RCVS website also maintains up-to-date guidance and contact information for both students and practices: www.rcvs.org.uk/lifelong-learning/students/veterinary-students/extra-mural-studies-ems

Many universities also include intramural rotations (IMR) – placements arranged within the veterinary school's own hospitals, partner practices or teaching farms – allowing students to gain structured clinical experience in an academic environment before progressing to fully external placements.

Reflection and professional development

Throughout both stages, students are expected to record and reflect on their learning experiences using electronic logs or portfolios, aligned with the RCVS Day One Competences. This ensures that every graduate leaves veterinary school with the practical, professional and ethical skills required to enter clinical practice safely and effectively.

Veterinary course types and entry routes

Veterinary medicine degrees in the UK all lead to registration with the Royal College of Veterinary Surgeons (RCVS), but entry routes and course structures vary slightly between universities. Understanding these options will help you find the route that best matches your background and experience.

- **Standard entry (D100)**: the typical five-year degree leading to BVSc (Bachelor of Veterinary Science) or BVMS (Bachelor of Veterinary Medicine and Surgery). This is the standard route for school-leavers with A levels (or equivalent) in science subjects.
- **Gateway or Foundation routes (D190/preliminary year)**: designed for students who show strong potential but may not meet the standard academic entry requirements. These courses often include an extra preparatory year focusing on biological sciences, chemistry and professional skills, before joining the main cohort.
- **Graduate entry**: some veterinary schools (such as Bristol, Surrey and RVC) offer accelerated or alternative-entry routes for graduates with relevant degrees (usually in biological or animal sciences). These programmes recognise prior learning but still provide full RCVS accreditation upon graduation.

- **Intercalated and combined degrees**: many veterinary schools allow students to take a year out to study for an additional BSc or MSc, often in areas such as pathology, pharmacology, animal behaviour or conservation medicine. These optional years are a chance to gain research experience or specialise early.

Diversity and widening access

Veterinary medicine has traditionally been one of the most competitive and academically demanding university subjects. However, UK veterinary schools and the Veterinary Schools Council (VSC) have made strong commitments to widening access and improving diversity within the profession.

Several universities now offer Gateway, contextual or widening participation routes to support talented applicants from underrepresented backgrounds, low-participation areas or non-traditional educational pathways. Examples include:

- Nottingham's Gateway to Veterinary Medicine (D190);
- RVC's Veterinary Gateway Programme (a one-year foundation course for widening-access applicants);
- Harper & Keele's contextual admissions policy, which considers applicants' educational and social circumstances.

Alongside these, national initiatives such as Vet Mentor, Vets: Stay, Go, Diversify and RCVS Diversity and Inclusion initiatives encourage inclusivity, representation and career support across all stages of veterinary education and practice.

Global recognition and accreditation

All veterinary degrees offered by UK universities must meet the professional standards set by the Royal College of Veterinary Surgeons (RCVS). Graduates from RCVS-accredited programmes are eligible to register as veterinary surgeons in the UK and to practise immediately upon graduation.

Several UK veterinary schools also hold additional international accreditations:

- **AVMA (American Veterinary Medical Association)**: enables graduates to practise in the United States and Canada (after passing national board exams).
- **EAEVE (European Association of Establishments for Veterinary Education)**: confirms that a degree meets the professional requirements to practise in Europe.
- **AVBC (Australasian Veterinary Boards Council)**: recognised in Australia and New Zealand.

These accreditations are reviewed regularly. For students considering working abroad, it's important to check the latest recognition status on the RCVS or Vet Schools Council websites before applying.

Notes on veterinary courses in the UK

Aberystwyth University (in partnership with the Royal Veterinary College)

Aberystwyth's veterinary school, delivered in partnership with the Royal Veterinary College, is the first to offer a veterinary degree in Wales. The course blends Aberystwyth's rural strengths with the RVC's world-class clinical facilities. Early years focus on animal science and husbandry, while later stages provide hands-on clinical training through the RVC's hospitals and partner practices.

- **Degree**: BVSc
- **Length**: five years (Years 1–2 in Aberystwyth; Years 3–5 at RVC Hawkshead)
- **Accreditation**: provisional RCVS status; full accreditation expected in 2026.
- **Course structure**: integrated curriculum progressing from healthy animal science to pathology, pharmacology and clinical practice.
- **Clinical training**: Years 3–5 at RVC hospitals and specialist centres.
- **EMS**: 12 weeks Animal Husbandry EMS and 26 weeks Clinical EMS (with 13 weeks in Wales).
- **Assessment**: exams, practical assessments and coursework.
- **Who it suits**: students interested in rural and production animal practice with access to large clinical resources.
- **Highlights**: combines Aberystwyth's agricultural expertise with RVC's clinical depth.

University of Bristol - Bristol Veterinary School

Bristol offers a dual-campus experience split between the city-based main campus and the rural Langford site. Teaching follows a spiral curriculum that builds from healthy animal science to clinical practice, with early practical exposure.

- **Degree**: BVSc Veterinary Science
- **Length**: five years
- **Accreditation**: RCVS, EAEVE, AVMA
- **Course structure**: systems-based curriculum integrating anatomy, physiology, disease mechanisms and clinical management.
- **Clinical training**: delivered at the Langford site through first-opinion and referral hospitals.

- **EMS**: 12 weeks Animal Husbandry EMS and 26 weeks Clinical EMS, including a period in a 'Foster Practice' for mentoring and continuity.
- **Assessment**: written exams, practical tests and group work.
- **Intercalation**: optional BSc after Year 3 or 4.
- **Who it suits**: students who like a mix of city life and rural clinical training.
- **Highlights**: hands-on from Year 1 with a lecture-free final year.

University of Cambridge - Department of Veterinary Medicine

Cambridge offers an academically rigorous six-year veterinary programme, combining deep scientific foundations with extensive clinical training supported by small-group supervisions.

- **Degree**: VetMB
- **Length**: six years
- **Accreditation**: RCVS (currently under review)
- **Course structure**: three pre-clinical years (with BA at the end of Year 3), followed by three clinical years.
- **Clinical training**: conducted at the Queen's Veterinary School Hospital, university farm and equine facilities.
- **EMS**: minimum of 12 weeks pre-clinical and around 26 weeks Clinical EMS.
- **Assessment**: written and practical exams, supervisions and continuous assessment.
- **Who it suits**: students seeking a research-intensive course with close academic support.
- **Highlights**: exceptionally strong scientific grounding and one of the most research-active UK vet schools.

Note: the RCVS has raised concerns about clinical caseload and facilities; accreditation status is currently under formal review.

University of Edinburgh - The Royal (Dick) School of Veterinary Studies

Edinburgh's Royal (Dick) School of Veterinary Studies offers a clinically integrated five-year programme at the Easter Bush campus, combining modern facilities with internationally recognised research links.

- **Degree**: BVM&S
- **Length**: five years
- **Accreditation**: RCVS, AVMA
- **Course structure**: integrated teaching from Day 1 with strong One Health and research themes.

- **Clinical training**: rotation-based, including small animal, equine and farm hospitals.
- **EMS**: completed in line with RCVS requirements.
- **Who it suits**: applicants interested in research-informed teaching with a blend of rural and university environments.
- **Highlights**: close links to the Roslin Institute and world-leading expertise in genetics and infectious disease.

University of Glasgow - School of Veterinary Medicine

Glasgow's BVMS programme combines tradition with international accreditation, offering a practical, problem-based curriculum.

- **Degree**: BVMS
- **Length**: five years
- **Accreditation**: RCVS, EAEVE, AVMA
- **Course structure**: three-phase curriculum covering foundational science, clinical training and professional development.
- **Clinical training**: delivered through university hospitals, Cochno Farm and external EMS.
- **EMS**: 12 weeks pre-clinical and 26 weeks clinical.
- **Intercalation**: optional after Year 3.
- **Who it suits**: students seeking strong global recognition and broad species exposure.
- **Highlights**: highly ranked in Europe with extensive clinical facilities.

Harper & Keele Veterinary School

Harper & Keele's collaborative programme combines strengths in agricultural science and clinical teaching, offering early practical exposure and a community-based veterinary education.

- **Degree**: BVetMS
- **Length**: five years
- **Accreditation**: fully RCVS accredited (2025)
- **Course structure**: spiral, clinically integrated curriculum with early animal handling and professional skills.
- **Clinical training**: delivered throughout via partner practices across species.
- **EMS**: 12 weeks AHEMS and 26 weeks CEMS; final year rotations are school-organised.
- **Assessment**: continuous assessment and competency sign-offs.
- **Who it suits**: students wanting a hands-on, vocational course with strong links to practice.
- **Highlights**: emphasis on workplace-based learning and preparation for real-world practice.

University of Lancashire - School of Veterinary Medicine

Lancashire's new veterinary programme focuses on early clinical contact, regional partnerships and preparation for roles in rural and mixed practice.

- **Degree**: BVMS
- **Length**: five years
- **Accreditation**: working towards full RCVS accreditation (expected 2028)
- **Course structure**: clinically integrated from Year 1, progressing to diagnostics, communication and professional practice.
- **Clinical training**: early practice exposure plus a 28-week final year placement, largely funded.
- **EMS**: 12 weeks AHEMS and 26 weeks CEMS, supported by a dedicated placement team.
- **Assessment**: written, practical and reflective assessments.
- **Who it suits**: applicants wanting a modern, community-oriented programme.
- **Highlights**: strong regional ties and emphasis on employability.

University of Liverpool - School of Veterinary Science

Liverpool combines urban teaching with rural clinical experience across its city campus and the Leahurst site, offering broad exposure across species.

- **Degree**: BVSc
- **Length**: five years
- **Accreditation**: RCVS, EAEVE, AVMA
- **Course structure**: pre-clinical and para-clinical teaching in Liverpool, followed by intensive clinical years at Leahurst.
- **Clinical training**: equine, farm and small animal hospitals, with strong links to Chester Zoo and regional farms.
- **EMS**: 12 weeks AHEMS and 26 weeks CEMS, with compulsory species-specific blocks (e.g. lambing, dairy, horses, poultry).
- **Assessment**: exams, practicals and clinical evaluations.
- **Intercalation**: optional BSc/MSc between Years 3 and 4.
- **Who it suits**: students seeking varied clinical experience and strong research integration.
- **Highlights**: exceptional equine, farm and wildlife experience.

Royal Veterinary College (RVC), University of London

The RVC is the UK's oldest and largest vet school, with an internationally recognised degree and world-leading clinical facilities.

2| Studying Veterinary Medicine

- **Degree**: BVetMed
- **Length**: five years
- **Accreditation**: RCVS, EAEVE, AVMA, AVBC
- **Course structure**: systems-based curriculum with early animal management at Camden and clinical years at Hawkshead.
- **Clinical training**: delivered at major referral hospitals including the Queen Mother Hospital for Animals and the Equine Referral Hospital.
- **EMS**: 12 weeks AHEMS and 26 weeks CEMS, recorded via the RCVS Student Experience Log.
- **Assessment**: OSCEs, DOPS, written tests and case-based evaluation.
- **Intercalation**: optional BSc in areas such as pathology, behaviour or bioveterinary science.
- **Who it suits**: students seeking an internationally focused programme with strong research and clinical depth.
- **Highlights**: exceptional facilities and global accreditation.

University of Nottingham - School of Veterinary Medicine and Science

Nottingham offers a modern, research-driven curriculum with early clinical exposure and an emphasis on applied learning.

- **Degree**: BVM BVS with BVMedSci
- **Length**: five years
- **Accreditation**: RCVS, EAEVE, AVMA
- **Course structure**: problem-based, clinically integrated curriculum. Students complete a compulsory research project leading to the BVMedSci at the end of Year 3.
- **Clinical training**: delivered through early exposure, intramural rotations and strong partner-practice links.
- **EMS**: 12 weeks AHEMS and 26 weeks CEMS, including 6 weeks of school-organised placements.
- **Assessment**: exams, practical tests, OSCEs and research-based coursework.
- **Intercalation**: embedded via the BVMedSci year.
- **Who it suits**: students who prefer structured teaching, early hands-on work and strong pastoral support.
- **Highlights**: high student satisfaction and employability with a clear, modern curriculum.

Scotland's Rural College (SRUC), Aberdeen

SRUC's new veterinary school, developed with the University of Aberdeen, focuses on livestock, rural practice and One Health through a distributed teaching model.

- **Degree**: BVMS
- **Length**: five years
- **Accreditation**: working towards full RCVS approval (expected 2029)
- **Course structure**: emphasis on rural mixed practice, sustainability and early clinical exposure.
- **Clinical training**: delivered via partner practices and agricultural enterprises across Scotland.
- **EMS**: 12 weeks AHEMS and 26 weeks CEMS.
- **Who it suits**: students interested in farm, mixed or rural practice.
- **Highlights**: first new Scottish vet school in over a century, designed to address rural veterinary shortages.

University of Surrey – School of Veterinary Medicine

Surrey offers a modern veterinary degree built around One Health, delivered through strong clinical partnerships rather than a single teaching hospital.

- **Degree**: BVMSci
- **Length**: five years
- **Accreditation**: fully RCVS accredited
- **Course structure**: systems-based curriculum with early handling, professional skills and optional research opportunities.
- **Clinical training**: delivered through an extensive partner-practice network covering small animal, equine, farm and public health.
- **EMS**: 12 weeks AHEMS and 26 weeks CEMS, supported by the placement office.
- **Assessment**: written and practical assessments, OSCEs and competency-based evaluation.
- **Intercalation**: opportunities in microbiology, infectious disease or One Health.
- **Who it suits**: students wanting a partnership-led, modern programme with strong research links.
- **Highlights**: purpose-built facilities and a curriculum rooted in One Health and sustainability.

Reminder: RCVS EMS requirement: All UK veterinary students must complete a minimum of 12 weeks of Animal Husbandry EMS (AHEMS) during the pre-clinical years and 26 weeks of Clinical EMS (CEMS) before final examinations. These placements are compulsory for RCVS registration and are designed to develop practical skills, professional confidence and an understanding of the veterinary workplace.

Fact: Cows can sleep standing up, but they can only dream lying down.

3 | Separating the sheep from the goats
Preparation and experience

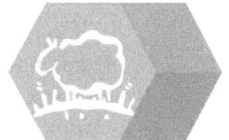

Becoming a veterinary surgeon is a long-term commitment that demands perseverance, focus and genuine motivation. Even with excellent grades and a strong application, it will take five to six years of intensive study and training before you can qualify and register as a vet. It's a journey that begins well before university, often years in advance, and success depends on careful preparation as well as academic achievement. Many students find it hard to look beyond their next test or practical during the sixth form, but veterinary schools are looking for more than just strong grades. They want evidence of long-term commitment, curiosity and hands-on experience that shows you truly understand what the profession involves.

Starting early

Ideally, your interest in animals and their welfare – in short, your commitment – should begin well before you submit your UCAS application. The most successful applicants show a long-standing curiosity about animals and a willingness to learn through experience, whether that means volunteering locally, caring for pets or exploring animal health through reading and online resources.

An interest in veterinary medicine can be sparked in many ways, through caring for pets, volunteering with animal charities or simply being inspired by documentaries and TV series that show the reality of animal care. Popular programmes such as *The Supervet*, *Mountain Vets* and *The Yorkshire Vet* offer a glimpse into the variety and emotional rewards of the profession.

Many successful applicants start gaining experience gradually, often by volunteering at weekends or during school holidays. This might involve helping at kennels, animal rescue centres, farms or stables – any environment where you can observe animal behaviour and learn what daily animal care really involves. Cleaning out enclosures or feeding animals might not sound glamorous, but these are the foundations of practical animal handling and demonstrate reliability and commitment.

If you have access to a local farm or similar setting, try to observe and ask questions. Curiosity and awareness are key: why is a calf coughing, what medication is being given, how do you recognise when an animal is unwell? Showing that you think critically about what you see will make your experience far more meaningful.

Not everyone discovers their ambition to be a vet early in life, and that's perfectly fine. What matters most is how you use the time you do have. Even if you're deciding later, careful planning and persistence can help you meet the work experience requirements that each UK veterinary school expects. What admissions tutors value most is not how early you started, but how much you learnt from the opportunities available to you.

Getting more experience

Once you've had some early exposure to animals, it's important to build on that experience by spending time in a veterinary setting. This isn't just to meet university requirements – it's also a chance to test your motivation and make sure this is truly the right path for you. The reality of veterinary work can be challenging, but it's also incredibly rewarding, and seeing it first-hand is the best way to understand what the profession involves.

When you're still at school or college, most placements will focus on observation and support rather than direct involvement in consultations. Many students begin by shadowing veterinary nurses or assisting with basic animal care and clinic preparation. These placements teach you valuable lessons about teamwork, communication and animal handling, and they also give you a realistic picture of the daily demands of veterinary life.

Some parts of animal care can be messy or emotionally difficult, and that's okay. What matters most is how you respond: staying calm, respectful and willing to help.

Work experience also helps you understand the profession's full scope, from preventative healthcare and client communication to ethical decision-making and public health. It's an essential part of your preparation and a key component of every veterinary school's entry criteria. More importantly, it helps you confirm that your enthusiasm for animal care extends beyond your own pets, and that you're ready for the practical and emotional realities of the job.

Specific university requirements

Here are some of the current expectations across UK veterinary schools. Always check the university's website for the most recent guidance.

- **Aberystwyth University** requires applicants to complete at least 140 hours of work experience before applying – 70 hours in one or more veterinary practices, and 70 hours in animal-related, non-clinical environments such as farms, kennels or rescue centres. At least half of the non-clinical experience must involve large animals, excluding horse riding or family-owned livestock. All experience must be completed within the 18 months prior to application, and applicants are also required to submit the Royal Veterinary College's Work Experience Applicant Summary Form as part of their application.
- The **University of Bristol** no longer specifies a fixed minimum number of hours for veterinary-related work experience. Instead, applicants complete a Supplementary Assessment Questionnaire (SAQ) that explores their experiences, insight into the profession and personal attributes. While placements in a veterinary practice or animal-related setting are encouraged, the focus is on the quality of reflection and understanding, rather than meeting a strict hours target.
- The **University of Cambridge** does not impose a fixed minimum number of hours of veterinary work experience. Instead, it recommends around two weeks (about 10–12 days) of relevant placement, either observing practice in a veterinary setting or working with animals in a commercial or charity environment.
- The **University of Edinburgh** veterinary medicine course does not specify a minimum number of days or weeks of work experience. Instead, applicants are encouraged to gain as broad and varied an experience as possible, covering veterinary practice, large and small animals, farms, kennels, zoos, abattoirs and labs. Applicants must also complete and submit a Work Experience Summary (WES) form by the specified deadline.
- The **University of Glasgow** does not set a formal minimum for work experience, but applicants are encouraged to complete at least one week in a veterinary practice to gain insight into the realities of the profession. The admissions team values a broad range of animal-handling experiences, including work with farm, small animal, equine or wildlife settings, and completion of virtual work experience courses where access to placements is limited. Most successful applicants typically complete between two and five weeks of relevant experience before applying. A short work experience form must also be submitted as part of the application process.

- **Harper & Keele** does not stipulate a fixed number of weeks for work experience. What they emphasise is meaningful, reflective exposure: applicants should spend time in veterinary practice and animal-related settings and be ready to discuss in detail what they observed and learnt. While some applicants may undertake two weeks in practice and additional weeks in non-clinical roles, the school recognises that opportunities vary and places greater weight on insight and maturity than on raw hours.
- The **University of Lancashire** does not require a specified minimum number of hours of work or animal experience for entry to its BVMS programme. Instead, applicants are encouraged to demonstrate relevant vocational experience – this might include time in a veterinary practice, farms, kennels or other animal-related settings, and reflect on what they have learnt. The admissions guidance emphasises quality, such as insight, motivation and understanding of the veterinary role, rather than a strict hours target.
- The **University of Liverpool** applicants must provide evidence of at least three weeks (15 working days) of relevant work experience obtained within the five years immediately preceding the application. At least one full week must be spent in a veterinary practice. If a student is unable to secure a week in a veterinary practice, they must instead complete a recognised virtual veterinary placement course (e.g. the 'Virtual Work Experience and Exploring the Veterinary Profession' MOOC) in addition to the 15 days of experience in other animal industry settings. Experience should involve work in a veterinary practice or the commercial animal industry (covering core species such as cattle, sheep, pigs, poultry, dogs, cats, rabbits); work solely with wildlife or zoo species is not included within this requirement. All experience must be documented via the university's designated portal, with detailed records of placement type, duration and signed verification from the provider.
- Applicants to the **University of Nottingham** must complete a minimum of five weeks' work experience. This must include at least three weeks' animal-handling experience (e.g. in a veterinary practice, kennels, cattery, zoo, wildlife park or research lab). Up to two weeks of the experience may instead come from customer-facing or teamwork roles (such as retail, sports team involvement) or completion of a virtual work experience course. The university requires that all work experience is completed within the three years before the application deadline.
- Applicants to the **Royal Veterinary College (RVC)** must complete at least 140 hours of relevant work experience, comprising 70 hours (two weeks) in one or more veterinary practices and a further 70 hours (two weeks) in animal-related environments such as farms, stables, kennels, animal shelters or zoos. All work experience must be completed within 18 months of the application deadline, though earlier placements can still be discussed in the application. The

RVC emphasises quality and reflection over quantity, encouraging applicants to think broadly about the role of vets in society. All applicants must also complete a Supplementary Work Experience Questionnaire to document their placements and provide brief reflections.
- **Scotland's Rural College** looks for evidence of recent and relevant practical experience, ideally including work in veterinary practice and/or large animal (farm/horse) settings, aligned with the school's rural and agricultural mission. There is no fixed minimum number of hours specified, but experience must be completed prior to interview and must demonstrate insight into the veterinary profession, animal health and welfare, and the applicant's ability to reflect on what they observed. Virtual work experience modules are accepted when physical placements are limited.
- Applicants to the **University of Surrey** veterinary medicine course are no longer required to complete formal veterinary practice placements as part of the shortlisting process. Instead, candidates are asked to complete an online questionnaire designed to assess insight into the profession, relevant personal attributes (such as communication, empathy, initiative) and understanding of current issues in veterinary medicine. While animal-related work experience is still encouraged, it is not mandatory for application.

Making the initial contact

Contacting a veterinary practice or farm to request work experience can feel intimidating, especially if you've never done it before. The key is to approach it with professionalism and clarity.

Practices prefer to hear directly from you rather than from a parent or teacher, as this demonstrates initiative and maturity – two qualities that admissions tutors also look for. Keep your message short, polite and purposeful. Introduce yourself, explain that you're considering a degree in veterinary medicine, and outline when you're available for a short placement. If relevant, mention any prior experience, and thank them for their time.

If you don't receive a reply, follow up courteously after a week or two. Many practices are busy, and persistence (when handled professionally) reflects well on you. Your school or college may also have lists of previous placement providers, and local vets or farmers can often point you towards other contacts. Building connections like this – networking – is an important part of working within the veterinary community.

Ultimately, securing work experience is your responsibility. Showing initiative, good communication skills and perseverance will help you stand out, both now and later in your career.

> **Example email**
>
> **Subject:** Work Experience Enquiry – Prospective Veterinary Student
>
> Dear [Dr/Mr/Ms Surname],
>
> My name is [Your Name], and I am a Year [12/13] student at [Your School/College]. I am planning to apply for veterinary medicine and would greatly value the opportunity to gain some work experience to learn more about life in practice.
>
> I am available between [insert dates] and would be happy to assist with any tasks appropriate for a student. Please let me know if this might be possible or if you require further details.
>
> Many thanks for your time and consideration.
>
> Kind regards,
> [Your Name]
> [Your Contact Details]

What to expect from a veterinary placement

Each veterinary practice is different, and so is each placement. Some vets are understandably cautious about taking on students they haven't met before – not because they don't want to help, but because supervising a placement requires time, preparation and responsibility for your safety. It's common for practices to suggest a short introductory visit before committing to a longer placement. This helps both you and the practice decide whether it's the right fit.

What you'll be asked to do will depend on the practice. In a small animal clinic, you might observe consultations, assist the veterinary nurses with cleaning, restocking and animal handling or help maintain the kennels. In a mixed or large animal practice, you could accompany vets on farm calls, learn about biosecurity procedures or assist with routine herd checks. Every experience offers insight into a different side of the profession.

Practices also vary in size and focus. Urban clinics may see mostly companion animals, while rural practices are often centred on farm and equine work. Wherever you go, enthusiasm, curiosity and professionalism will leave a positive impression.

Making a positive impression in practice

Vets and veterinary nurses quickly notice how students behave during placements. The most successful students treat every task, from cleaning to observing consultations, as an opportunity to learn.

Here are some of the qualities that practices look for:

- **Willingness to help**: get involved wherever possible. Cleaning kennels or preparing equipment may not be glamorous, but it's essential and demonstrates teamwork.
- **Observation skills**: watch closely how procedures are carried out, from taking blood samples to bandaging, and think about why each step is done the way it is.
- **Professionalism and appearance**: keep your clothing neat, follow hygiene rules and always be mindful of clients' perceptions.
- **Communication**: be polite, approachable and attentive to both staff and clients. A friendly, professional manner leaves a lasting impression.
- **Curiosity**: ask thoughtful questions when appropriate, especially about cases, techniques or ethical decisions. This shows genuine engagement.
- **Empathy**: pay attention to how vets speak with owners about difficult situations. You'll learn as much from these conversations as from clinical procedures.

Every placement is an opportunity to practise these skills. How you approach your work experience can reveal a lot about your potential as a future vet.

Building your experience portfolio

There's no single route to gaining experience before applying to veterinary school – every student's journey looks different. What matters is that you explore a variety of settings, reflect on what you've learnt, and show genuine curiosity about animal health and welfare.

Here are some examples of valuable experiences to consider:

- **Veterinary practices**: try to gain experience in both small animal and, if possible, large animal or mixed practices. Even short placements can help you understand how different practices operate.
- **Animal husbandry**: work with livestock on farms, assist during lambing or milking or help at riding stables to learn about equine care and management.
- **Animal welfare and charities**: volunteer with organisations such as the RSPCA, PDSA, Blue Cross, Dogs Trust or local rescue centres. This can help you understand welfare, rehoming and owner education.
- **Laboratories and research**: spend time in a laboratory setting, shadow a technician or explore veterinary public health and One Health topics through online courses or university outreach programmes.
- **Wildlife and conservation**: opportunities at zoos, wildlife rehabilitation centres or conservation projects can give you insight into exotic and wild animal medicine.

- **Virtual experiences**: many veterinary schools recognise online placements such as the *Virtual Work Experience and Exploring the Veterinary Profession* course developed by the University of Nottingham and FutureLearn.
- **Community or educational work**: helping with public-facing animal events, educational talks or pet-care workshops can develop your communication and teamwork skills.

Remember, quality and reflection matter more than quantity. Admissions tutors are interested in what you learnt, how the experience influenced your understanding of the profession and how it strengthened your motivation to apply.

Case study

James grew up around animals and has always taken a hands-on approach to rearing and looking after them, even getting his own sheep! Although animals have always been a part of his life, he initially started along a different career trajectory before reflecting on his experiences and committing to veterinary medicine.

'I chose to study veterinary medicine so that I could work with animals. I have always had an interest in the care and husbandry of animals, whether that be pets or large farm animals. I was lucky enough to grow up around dogs and cats and large animals such as cows, sheep and ponies. I am really excited to be studying veterinary medicine to continue my journey learning about companion and farm animals and how to treat them. I also enjoy working with people as well, which is important as vets need to be able to communicate well with the animal owners.

'Before applying, I undertook a range of work-experience placements, including one week at a large animal vets, two weeks at two small animal clinics, one week at a riding stables, three days with a beef farmer, one day with a shepherd, one week with a farrier and two weeks on a dairy farm.

'Working at small-animal clinics, I was able to follow the day-to-day aspects of the job, such as consultations, vaccinations, spays and neuters. One particular case that fascinated me was a Bichon Frise with chylothorax, where I helped to drain the fluid from the thoracic cavity twice. I saw the dexterity and diagnostic skills required to locate the fluid using an ultrasound scanner and a needle. Seeing emergency cases where the vets did all they could, but ultimately, it was kinder to euthanise the animal, highlighted to me the skills required to work in high-pressure situations and to communicate sensitively with emotional owners. While watching a post-mortem on a Rottweiler, I was able to handle some of the tissues and apply my biological knowledge to identify various parts of the anatomy.

'Experience with large animal vets allowed me to see routine work, such as scanning cows on dairy farms, TB testing and working with farmers to create herd health plans. Helping with TB testing by recording the results of the test and assisting in the successful calving of a Highland cow demonstrated the necessity of good communication skills when working with other vets and the farmers.

'Initially I studied A levels in Maths, Geography and Physics, as well as completed an EPQ and secured good grades (AAB and an A* respectively). I originally pursued mechanical engineering at the University of Nottingham, but not long after I started this degree, I realised that it was veterinary medicine that I really wanted to do. Before making any rash decisions, I undertook work experience with my local farm vets during the Christmas break. This experience made me confident that I would be making the right decision by leaving the engineering course and I went back to college to study A levels in Chemistry and Biology in one year, which was tough, but I got A grades and met my offer for vet school.

'I am now in my first year of veterinary medicine at the University of Nottingham. The course is fantastic. As overwhelming as veterinary school is at first, I am enjoying the content and the work with animals. Some people find aspects of the course, such as dissection, quite daunting, but it's actually really interesting being able to relate what we have learned in lectures to the cadavers. I prefer working with large animals compared to small animals, though!

'In the future, I hope to practise as a farm vet or as a vet in a mixed practice. However, there is still plenty of time left for me to change my mind! My advice for aspiring vets during the application is don't be too hard on yourself, as it is a well-known fact that veterinary medicine is one of the most competitive courses to get onto.'

Variety and commitment

Veterinary schools value applicants who have gained experience across a variety of settings and who have shown sustained commitment over time. Seeing different aspects of veterinary work, such as small animal practice, farms, equine work and animal welfare organisations, helps you understand the breadth of the profession and shows that you've taken the time to explore your interest fully.

Try to gain experience in more than one type of environment, even if some placements are short. A single day in a small animal practice and another in a mixed practice can still be valuable if you approach each with curiosity and reflect on what you've learnt.

Just as important as variety is commitment. Admissions tutors are often impressed by applicants who return to the same placement or stay involved with an organisation over several months. This shows reliability, enthusiasm and the ability to build trust with professionals – qualities that are highly valued in veterinary medicine.

Don't worry if you can't access every type of placement. What matters most is making the most of the opportunities available to you, showing perseverance and demonstrating that you've taken time to understand the realities of the job.

Getting the most out of your work experience

Work experience isn't just a requirement for your veterinary application – it's your chance to find out whether this career is truly right for you. It's about testing your motivation, learning from real professionals and gaining insight into the rewards and challenges of working with animals and their owners.

You may discover that parts of veterinary medicine you expected to enjoy aren't what you imagined, or that an unexpected area sparks new enthusiasm. Whether you're cleaning kennels, shadowing consultations or assisting on a farm, every placement offers valuable lessons if you approach it with curiosity, professionalism and an open mind.

Make the most of your experience by:

- **Keeping a reflective journal**: write short notes after each day or placement about what you did, what you learnt and how it made you feel. Record both positive and challenging moments – reflection shows growth.
- **Noticing what stands out**: think about what you enjoyed, what surprised you and what you found difficult. These observations will help you identify your strengths and areas for development.
- **Talking to everyone**: ask questions – not just of the vets, but also veterinary nurses, receptionists and other staff. Each plays a vital role in how the practice runs.
- **Engaging with owners**: notice how vets communicate with clients, particularly in sensitive situations. How would you handle similar conversations?
- **Being flexible**: some placements are harder to secure due to biosecurity rules or limited availability. If a placement falls through, try to find another in a different animal setting – shelters, stables or wildlife centres can all provide valuable insights.

Reflecting on what you learn

Keeping a short reflective journal can help you understand what you're learning and prepare for your personal statement or interviews.

3| Preparation and Experience

You might include:

- **What you did**: the setting, your role and whom you worked with.
- **What you learnt**: new knowledge, techniques or professional behaviours.
- **Skills you observed**: such as teamwork, communication or empathy.
- **Your reflections**: what did you find rewarding, challenging or surprising? How did this experience influence your decision to study veterinary medicine?

Reflection doesn't have to be lengthy or formal – a few bullet points in a notebook or phone app can be enough. What matters most is that you take time to think about what each experience has taught you about the realities of veterinary medicine and about yourself.

TIP!

Try using the simple *What? So what? Now what?* model. Ask yourself what happened, why it mattered and how it might shape your future actions or goals.

Example reflection entry

Placement: small animal veterinary practice, one-week placement

Day: 3

What?

I observed several consultations, including a dog with a recurring ear infection and a cat being vaccinated. I also helped prepare the consultation rooms between appointments and watched a spay surgery.

So what?

I realised how much time vets spend communicating with owners, not just treating animals. The vet explained the cat's vaccination plan clearly and reassured a nervous owner – it showed how vital empathy and communication are. I also noticed how calm and methodical the team were in surgery, which helped me understand how important teamwork and attention to detail are in clinical settings.

Now what?

This experience confirmed that I enjoy the mix of practical and people-focused work in veterinary medicine. I want to develop my communication skills further, perhaps by volunteering with an animal charity where I can talk to owners about pet care.

Online work experience

In recent years, many veterinary schools have begun to recognise online work experience programmes as a valuable way to learn about the profession, particularly for applicants who may find it difficult to access traditional placements. These courses complement hands-on experience by helping you explore the wide range of roles and responsibilities within veterinary medicine, and reflect on what skills and values the profession requires.

A widely recommended option is the Virtual Work Experience and Exploring the Veterinary Profession course, hosted by FutureLearn and developed by the University of Nottingham in collaboration with all UK veterinary schools. It offers interactive case studies, videos and activities that introduce you to real veterinary scenarios and ethical decision-making. Completing it demonstrates motivation, insight and a proactive approach to learning – qualities that admissions tutors value highly.

You can find the course by searching 'Vet School Application Support FutureLearn' on the FutureLearn website.

Beyond work experience

Your preparation for veterinary school shouldn't stop at work experience. The best applicants also show curiosity about wider issues in animal health, research and the profession as a whole. Exploring veterinary medicine beyond formal placements helps you demonstrate genuine motivation and independent learning – two qualities that admissions tutors value highly.

- **Stay informed**: keep up to date with current issues in veterinary practice and animal health. This might include new disease outbreaks, animal welfare legislation or debates around sustainability and antimicrobial resistance. Following reputable sources such as the British Veterinary Association (BVA), Vet Record, or news stories from the RCVS will help you build awareness of the context in which vets work.
- **Keep learning independently**: veterinary medicine is a lifelong learning profession. Showing that you've taken the initiative to explore topics independently, such as through online courses, podcasts or TED Talks, demonstrates intellectual curiosity and commitment. Platforms like FutureLearn often host short, free courses on animal health and science that can enrich your understanding and provide examples to discuss in interviews.

- **Engage with the wider community**: social media can offer valuable insights into the realities of veterinary life. Many vets and students share their experiences through YouTube, Instagram and blogs. While these platforms can be informal, following credible accounts can help you understand the challenges and rewards of the profession, and show that you're actively engaging with the community you hope to join.

> **TIP!**
>
> Keeping a short log of articles, podcasts or online talks you've explored can be useful for interview preparation. Reflect on what you learnt and how it shaped your view of the veterinary profession.

> **Fact**: Hummingbirds are the only birds capable of sustained backward flight, thanks to their unique ability to rotate their wings in a full figure-eight motion.

4| The 'Jack Russell' group
Choosing your course

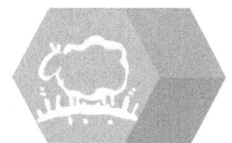

Getting into veterinary school takes more than enthusiasm for animals – it requires careful preparation and an informed understanding of what each course involves. With only a limited number of veterinary schools in the UK, it's vital to research your options thoroughly and to reflect on what type of course and environment will suit you best. The more time you invest in understanding how each programme is structured, the better your application, and the smoother your transition into university life will be.

Choice of school

Once you've completed your work experience and confirmed that veterinary medicine is the path for you, the next step is to research your choice of veterinary school thoroughly. With so few schools in the UK, every choice counts. When comparing universities, consider:

- how the course is structured and the teaching styles used;
- the academic and admissions requirements;
- the location and type of university environment;
- opportunities such as intercalation, research or placements abroad.

Finding reliable information

The best place to start is the UCAS website (www.ucas.com), which lists all accredited UK veterinary degrees and links directly to university websites. Each veterinary school publishes detailed guidance on entry requirements, work experience expectations and course structure, but these details can change from year to year, so always check again before applying.

If you can't find the information you need online, don't hesitate to contact the admissions office or veterinary school directly by email. Asking clear, polite questions shows genuine interest and initiative.

> **TIP!**
>
> Many universities offer several routes into veterinary medicine, including Gateway or Foundation years and graduate-entry programmes. Make sure you're reading the details for the correct course.

Open days

Attending open days is one of the best ways to explore what a veterinary school is really like. You'll have the chance to tour teaching facilities, meet lecturers and current students and get a sense of the campus environment. Because you'll be spending five years or more there, it's important to find somewhere that feels right for you, both academically and personally.

Information about open days is available on university websites or at www.opendays.com. Many events include bookable talks or sample lectures, so register early to secure your place.

If you can't make an official open day, contact the admissions team to see if a smaller visit or departmental tour is possible. Even walking around the main campus informally can help you picture yourself living and studying there.

Most universities now also offer virtual open days, which let you explore courses remotely through live Q&As, recorded talks and virtual tours. While they don't replace the experience of visiting in person, they're a great way to compare more universities in a short space of time, without the cost or travel.

Virtual open days often include online chats with current students and lecturers, so have your questions ready. You could ask about what a typical week looks like, how clinical teaching is structured or what support is available for placements.

League tables

University league tables can give you an overview of student satisfaction, research quality and graduate prospects, but they only tell part of the story. All UK veterinary schools are accredited by the Royal College of Veterinary Surgeons (RCVS), meaning that graduates from each can practise as vets in the UK.

League tables can vary depending on the data used, so use them as a starting point, not the deciding factor. Think instead about which course structure, teaching style and location will help *you* thrive.

Table 1 Complete University Guide veterinary school rankings 2026

Veterinary School	Rank
University of Cambridge	1
University of Liverpool	2
University of Nottingham	3
University of Surrey	4
University of Glasgow	5
Royal Veterinary College, University of London	6
University of Edinburgh	7
University of Bristol	8
Harper and Keele Veterinary School	9

Source: www.thecompleteuniversityguide.co.uk/league-tables/rankings/veterinary-medicine. Reprinted with kind permission from the Complete University Guide (www.thecompleteuniversityguide).

Course entry requirements

The academic entry requirements for veterinary medicine are broadly similar across UK vet schools, but there are some key differences. It's essential to check the most up-to-date information before making your choices, as entry criteria, subject requirements and contextual (widening participation) policies are reviewed regularly.

All UK veterinary schools now have widening participation policies, meaning they may make slightly lower offers for students from specific backgrounds, schools or regions, or for those who have faced educational disadvantage. Make sure to check whether you are eligible for these schemes when researching your options.

In addition, many universities offer alternative routes into veterinary medicine, such as Gateway or Foundation pathways and pre-clinical courses. These are designed for students who have the potential to succeed in veterinary medicine but may not yet meet the standard entry requirements, or who need extra preparation before starting the main degree. Always confirm that you are reviewing the correct course when checking entry criteria.

You can find reliable information about entry requirements from the following sources:

- individual university websites (the most accurate and frequently updated source);
- the UCAS website – www.ucas.com;
- university prospectuses or online brochures;
- university admissions teams, who can answer questions about eligibility or qualifications;

- HEAP 2027: University Degree Course Offers by Brian Heap (Trotman), which provides a comparative overview of entry grades.

Typical entry offers for the 2024–25 admissions cycle are shown in Table 2 on the following pages.

Academic and subject requirements

What admissions tutors look for

Veterinary medicine is one of the most competitive degree subjects in the UK, so universities will look carefully at your academic background. Admissions tutors consider your GCSE results, A level subjects and predicted grades and any extenuating circumstances that might have affected your performance.

Most successful applicants have strong GCSEs, typically grades 7–9 (A–A*), particularly in English language, mathematics, biology and chemistry. While most vet schools ask for a minimum of grade 6 (B) in these subjects, exact requirements vary – always check the university's admissions pages for the most accurate information.

If you have mitigating circumstances (e.g. illness or family issues) that affected your performance, ask your referee to mention this clearly in your UCAS reference, and contact the university for guidance on whether additional evidence is needed.

Choosing your A levels

All UK veterinary schools require chemistry at A level, and almost all also require biology. Your third subject is usually flexible – many students choose another science or maths (such as physics, mathematics or further mathematics), but subjects like psychology, geography or even a humanities subject are also accepted. The key is to choose subjects you enjoy and can excel in.

You'll typically need AAA at A level, although some schools – including Aberystwyth, Bristol, Harper & Keele and the RVC – make contextual offers of AAB or ABB for widening participation candidates.

When selecting your subjects, consider three key points:

1. **Play to your strengths**: choose subjects where you are confident you can achieve high grades.
2. **Stay relevant**: prioritise subjects that will help with your veterinary studies, especially biology and chemistry.
3. **Broaden your interests**: a contrasting third subject can make you stand out, showing balance and wider curiosity.

Table 2 Typical student offers 2024–25

University	Preferred Grades	Access Course Available	Access Course Accepted	Subjects Required	BTEC Accepted
Aberystwyth	AAA at A level, including biology and chemistry. Contextual offers typically ABB (with an A in biology or chemistry). IB: 6, 6, 6 at Higher Level including biology and chemistry. GCSEs: Five at grade 7 including science (Double Award or biology and chemistry), plus grade 6 in English language, mathematics and physics (if taken separately).	No specific internal 'Gateway' or Foundation programme. However, applicants with a QAA-recognised science-based Access to HE Diploma are considered.	Yes – science-based Access to HE Diploma with at least 15 Level 3 credits at Distinction in biology and 15 Level 3 credits at Distinction in chemistry, and all remaining Level 3 credits at Merit or above. The Birkbeck Certificate of Higher Education in Subjects Allied to medicine is also accepted if Distinctions are achieved in biology and chemistry modules.	Biology and chemistry at grade A/Higher Level 6.	Yes – science-based Extended Diploma is accepted at D*D overall, with Distinctions in required science units.
Bristol	AAA at A level (including chemistry and one of biology, physics, mathematics or further mathematics). Contextual offer ABB (including A in chemistry and one of the other required subjects). IB: approx. 36 points including 6,6 at Higher Level in chemistry and one of biology, physics or mathematics.	Yes – the University offers a Gateway to Veterinary Science (D108) route for students from widening participation backgrounds.	Yes – science-based Access to HE Diplomas are accepted. The university's Access policy states that relevant Access qualifications in 'Sciences, Biomedical/Medical/Health Sciences or similar' are eligible, and the standard offer includes D:30 credits and M:15 credits for Access to HE.	Chemistry plus one of biology, physics and mathematics or further mathematics (including A level science practical passes).	Yes – A BTEC Level 3 National Extended Diploma is listed in the course data as acceptable with grade DDD.
Cambridge	A*AA at A level (chemistry plus one of biology, physics or mathematics). IB: 41–42 points overall.	No formal Gateway or Foundation course listed.	Not standard; individual college discretion.	Chemistry plus one of biology, physics or mathematics.	No standard acceptance published; applicants should check college-specific requirements.

(Continued)

Table 2 (Continued)

University	Preferred Grades	Access Course Available	Access Course Accepted	Subjects Required	BTEC Accepted
Edinburgh	AAA at A level, including chemistry and biology (or human biology), plus one other approved subject. Widening-access offers are typically AAB with chemistry (A) and biology/human biology (A). IB: 38 points overall with Higher Level 6,6,6 in chemistry, biology and a third subject (widening-access: 36 points).	No distinct Gateway/Foundation route listed for standard entry; school-leavers meeting the academic criteria apply.	SWAP (Scottish Wider Access Programme) considered for mature/adult applicants who meet eligibility; AAA-pass in mathematics, biology and chemistry is required to be considered.	Chemistry plus biology (or human biology) plus one other University-approved subject at A level.	Not standardly listed as accepted for the five-year entry route; applicants should consult the school for guidance.
Glasgow	AAA at A level, including biology and chemistry. IB: 38 points overall (HL 6,6,6) including biology and chemistry.	Yes – adult/Access pathways exist (e.g. Access to Medical Studies) though not a standard Gateway for veterinary entry.	No standard Access/Foundation route acceptance published; applicants should check with admissions.	A levels: biology and chemistry (grade A) plus another approved subject.	No – BTEC National Extended Diploma not accepted for this programme.
Harper & Keele	AAA at A level (A in biology or chemistry; A in a second science subject; A in a third subject). IB: 6, 6, 6 HL including biology or chemistry and a second science.	Yes – Year 0/Foundation options (Veterinary Bioscience with Access to Veterinary Medicine) and transfer routes from related animal-science degrees.	Yes – science-based Diplomas or Foundation Years (students must meet minimum pass criteria and subsequent progression).	Biology or chemistry at A level (grade A) plus a second science subject (biology, chemistry, physics, maths, further maths or statistics) at grade A; third subject at grade A.	Yes – BTEC Level 3 National Extended Diploma at DDD (science/animal-management related) with required units in Animal Biology, Health & Diseases, Breeding & Genetics.
Lancashire	AAB at A level (two science subjects plus one other) or ABB (three science subjects, or two science subjects plus mathematics).	Yes – Foundation Year/Gateway route (BVMS with Foundation Entry).	Yes – details vary, e.g. Foundation Year requires BBB A levels or DDM BTEC for entry into the standard degree.	Science subjects required at A level: typically biology, chemistry, physics, mathematics or equivalents (two science subjects plus one other).	Yes – BTEC Extended Diploma (science/animal-management related) at DDD*.

Liverpool	AAA at A level (grade A in biology or human biology, grade A in chemistry). IB: 36 points overall including grade 6 HL biology and grade 6 HL chemistry.	Yes – a Foundation Year (Year 0) for mature or non-traditional applicants leading into the BVSc.	Yes – applicants via the Foundation route may progress into the standard programme.	Biology (or human biology) and chemistry at A level (grade A). If chemistry is not taken at A level then AS grade B in chemistry plus another academic science subject at A level.	No – BTEC Level 3 National Extended Diploma is not accepted for entry to the standard BVSc programme.
Nottingham	AAB at A level (including biology and chemistry).	Yes – Gateway/Preliminary Year option (six-year version) for students who do not meet standard entry requirements.	Yes – progression from the Gateway/Preliminary Year into the standard course.	Chemistry and biology at A level (grade A) plus a third subject at required grade.	No – BTEC Level 3 National Extended Diploma is not accepted for the standard entry route.
London (RVC)	AAA at A level (including A in biology and A in chemistry, plus a third subject). Contextual offers typically ABB (with an A in biology or chemistry). IB: 6, 6, 6 at Higher Level including biology, chemistry and a third subject.	Yes – the 'Veterinary Gateway' preparatory year (UCAS code D190) for widening participation applicants.	Yes – science-based Access to HE Diploma accepted (minimum 15 L3 credits in biology at Distinction and 15 L3 credits in chemistry at Distinction).	Biology and chemistry at A level (grade A), and a third subject of your choice.	Yes – science-based Extended Diploma (applied science/ biomedical science/animal management (science)) at DDD* with required Distinctions in specified units.

(Continued)

Table 2 (Continued)

University	Preferred Grades	Access Course Available	Access Course Accepted	Subjects Required	BTEC Accepted
SRUC	Two Advanced Highers at BB (including one science) plus five Highers at AABBB (with at least two science subjects: chemistry, biology, physics, human biology or maths).	Yes – SRUC accepts a wide range of access-level and non-standard qualifications under its flexible entry policy.	Yes – Applications from those with non-standard qualifications or strong vocational experience may be considered; individual review required.	Science subjects at Higher/Advanced Higher Level (including at least two from chemistry, biology, physics, human biology or maths).	Not specified as a standard accepted qualification for this programme; applicants should contact SRUC admissions.
Surrey	AAA at A level, including A in biology and A in chemistry. IB: 35 points overall, including HL6 in biology and chemistry.	No formal Gateway/Foundation programme listed for the standard five-year veterinary course (applicants should confirm any alternative routes).	Yes – QAA-accredited Access to Higher Education Diploma with 45 Level 3 credits at Distinction, including 15 in biology at Distinction and 15 in chemistry at Distinction; the remaining 15 credits at Distinction can be in any subject. The Birkbeck University Certificate of Higher Education in Subjects Allied to medicine is also accepted with Distinction overall and Distinction in all biology and chemistry modules.	Biology and chemistry (grade A at A level). Pass required in science Practical Endorsement.	No – BTEC Level 3 National Extended Diploma is not accepted for veterinary medicine.

Taking four A levels

Some students start with four A levels, but there is no expectation or advantage in doing so. Veterinary schools make offers based on three subjects only, and the additional workload can make it harder to achieve top grades. If you do take four subjects in Year 12, you may wish to drop one before Year 13 to focus on quality rather than quantity.

Predicted grades and references

Your teachers' predicted grades are an important part of your UCAS application. These are usually based on your GCSE performance, classwork and Year 12 assessments. For this reason, it's vital to work consistently hard throughout Year 12 to secure strong predictions.

If there are reasons your earlier grades don't reflect your ability, such as illness, family circumstances or a disrupted learning period, make sure your referee knows, so they can include this in your reference. Universities will sometimes ask for additional supporting evidence, so it's best to be transparent from the outset.

Other qualifications

Scottish Highers

Applicants offering Scottish qualifications typically need AAAAA–AAABB at Higher Level, with Advanced Highers in chemistry and biology taken in the final year. Some universities encourage students to take a new subject at Higher Level if only two Advanced Highers are studied in the sixth year. Highers alone are generally not sufficient for entry to veterinary medicine.

Irish Leaving Certificate

The Irish Leaving Certificate is widely accepted. Applicants are usually expected to achieve at least H1, H1, H2, H2, H2, H2, including H1 grades in biology and/or chemistry. If physics is not taken at Leaving Certificate level, a high grade at Junior Certificate may be considered instead.

International Baccalaureate and European Baccalaureate

The IB is fully accepted by all UK veterinary schools. Students typically need 36–38 points overall, with 6,6,6 or 7,6,6 at Higher Level, including chemistry and biology. A third science or mathematics subject at either Higher or Standard Level is often recommended.

For the European Baccalaureate, most schools ask for an overall average of 80–88%, with strong performance in chemistry and biology.

Extended Project Qualification (EPQ)

The EPQ encourages independent learning and research – skills that are highly valued by universities. While it is not part of conditional offers, it can enhance an application, especially if your project explores a relevant topic such as animal welfare, zoonotic disease or sustainable farming. It may also provide useful discussion points at interview. However, ensure your EPQ does not detract from achieving strong A level grades, which remain the priority.

BTEC

BTEC qualifications are increasingly accepted, particularly in applied science or animal management. Universities such as the RVC, Bristol, Aberystwyth, Harper & Keele and UCLan consider BTEC applicants, often requiring high overall grades (typically DDD* or DDD) and, in some cases, an accompanying A level in chemistry or biology. Always check individual university websites, as requirements vary.

> **Note:** Each veterinary school sets its own entry criteria. Always refer to the most up-to-date information on university websites before applying.

Veterinary Gateway pathway

Gateway and Foundation programmes provide routes into veterinary medicine for applicants from widening participation backgrounds or those who do not meet the standard entry requirements. These courses combine academic support with skills development and progression to the full veterinary degree upon successful completion.

You may be eligible if you have attended a non-selective state school, are from a low-income household or are the first in your family to attend university. Some programmes also consider applicants who have faced educational disruption or who live in areas with low progression to higher education.

Currently, Gateway or Foundation courses are offered at the following veterinary schools:

- Bristol – Gateway to Veterinary Science (D108);
- Harper & Keele – Extended Degree Veterinary Bioscience (XD01);
- Nottingham – Veterinary Gateway (D190);
- Royal Veterinary College (RVC) – Veterinary Gateway Programme (D190).

Choosing the right veterinary school: a checklist

University is about more than just lectures and exams – it's an experience that will shape both your professional and personal life. Choosing the right veterinary school means thinking carefully about where and how you want to study, not just what grades you need.

You'll be spending at least five years on your degree, so make sure it's a place where you can picture yourself thriving. Consider both the academic environment and the lifestyle that comes with it.

Here are some key things to think about when making your decision:

- **Research every veterinary school carefully**: use university websites and the UCAS course search to find up-to-date information on entry requirements, course structure and special features.
- **Compare teaching styles and course content**: some schools are more problem-based or clinically integrated, while others focus more heavily on traditional lectures and theory in the early years.
- **Visit open days**, either in person or virtually, to explore facilities, meet students and staff and get a real sense of the learning environment.
- **Think about the setting**: would you prefer a city-based university like Bristol or Glasgow, or a self-contained rural campus like Nottingham or Harper & Keele?
- **Consider distance and cost**: how far will you be from home, and what are the living costs in that area? Remember that expenses such as accommodation, transport and EMS placements can add up.
- **Check practicalities**: if you don't drive, is the campus well-connected by public transport? This is especially important for travelling to EMS placements and clinical settings.
- **Explore the wider student experience**: look at sports, societies, welfare support and accommodation options – you'll want to enjoy your time outside the lecture theatre too.
- **Understand what each university looks for in applicants**: make sure you meet or are working towards the required grades and experience. If not, plan early to fill those gaps through work experience or additional study.
- **Review the course modules**: while all veterinary programmes are accredited by the RCVS, some have distinctive areas of focus such as research, global health or business and entrepreneurship.

The fifth choice

When applying through UCAS, you can make up to five course choices, but for veterinary medicine, you may apply to a maximum of four veterinary schools. This leaves you with one remaining fifth choice – a decision that deserves careful thought.

There are two main approaches to consider:

Leaving the fifth choice blank

If you are completely committed to becoming a vet and would not consider any other degree, you might prefer not to use your fifth choice. This avoids the need to balance two different course applications within your personal statement.

If you are unsuccessful, you can use the year ahead to strengthen your application by gaining further work experience, improving your grades or completing an additional qualification such as an Access course. Many students take a planned gap year for this purpose and are successful in the following cycle.

Applying for an alternative course

Alternatively, you may wish to use your fifth choice for a related degree, particularly if:

- you would like to go to university even if you don't secure a veterinary place this year;
- you are open to studying a related subject first, then applying to veterinary medicine as a graduate.

If you choose this route, aim for a scientifically related subject such as bioveterinary science, animal science, zoology or biological sciences. These degrees share similar content and can provide a strong foundation for a later graduate-entry application.

Because your UCAS personal statement can only be submitted once, it will focus on veterinary medicine. Admissions tutors for other courses will understand this, but it's polite to email the admissions office explaining your situation and expressing your genuine interest in the alternative course. Some universities may invite you to submit a short supplementary statement to outline your motivation for that subject.

Graduate-entry route: pros and cons

If you take an alternative BSc first, there are both advantages and disadvantages to consider.

Pros

- You will gain valuable scientific knowledge and laboratory skills relevant to veterinary study.
- Graduate applicants often bring maturity, focus and strong academic habits that strengthen their veterinary applications.
- Having both a BSc and a veterinary degree can enhance your long-term career prospects, especially in research, academia or public health.
- The experience helps you confirm whether veterinary medicine truly aligns with your interests and values.

Cons

- It adds at least three extra years of study, plus the additional cost of tuition and living expenses.
- Graduate-entry veterinary medicine is extremely competitive, with fewer places available.
- You may not be eligible for full student finance for a second undergraduate degree.
- If your first degree is unrelated, you might need to complete extra science prerequisites before applying.

Key takeaway:

Using your fifth choice can be a smart safety net if you choose a relevant subject that genuinely interests you. However, if veterinary medicine is your clear and only goal, it's equally valid to leave the space blank and focus on reapplying with a stronger application next year.

> **Fact**: A group of owls is called a parliament.

5 | Take the bull by the horns in the cattle market
The UCAS application

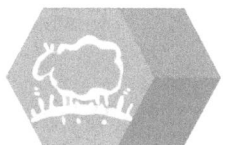

Gaining a place to study veterinary medicine is one of the most competitive challenges in higher education. Admissions tutors are not only looking for students with outstanding academic potential – they are also selecting future members of the veterinary profession. Their role is to identify applicants who combine strong scientific ability with motivation, resilience, empathy and a genuine commitment to animal welfare.

Although grades are an essential part of selection, motivation and personal qualities often distinguish successful applicants from equally able peers. Admissions tutors want to see evidence that you understand the realities of veterinary work, have reflected on your experiences and are prepared for both the rewards and the challenges of the career.

Every element of your application contributes to the overall impression you create. This includes your predicted grades and academic record, your school or college reference, your work and extracurricular experience and your personal statement – a crucial section where you explain why you want to study veterinary medicine and what makes you suited to it.

Applications for veterinary medicine are made through UCAS (Universities and Colleges Admissions Service). Most sections of the UCAS form are factual, including your qualifications, contact details and the four veterinary schools you are applying to, but the personal statement and reference give admissions tutors a deeper sense of who you are as a future vet.

Once your application has been submitted, universities will review it carefully to decide whether to invite you to interview. Most UK veterinary schools interview shortlisted candidates, typically through panel or multiple mini-interview (MMI) formats. The University of Bristol remains the only UK vet school that does not routinely interview, instead using its Supplementary Assessment Questionnaire (SAQ) as an alternative selection method.

What happens to your application?

By the 15 October UCAS deadline, veterinary schools receive far more applications than they have places available. Admissions teams must therefore make careful decisions about who progresses to the next stage of selection.

Most universities begin with a screening process, checking that applicants meet the required entry criteria – for example, the correct A level subjects, predicted grades (typically AAA or above) and minimum GCSE results. Applications that don't meet these basic requirements are normally rejected automatically, so it's essential to double-check that you qualify before you apply.

If you're unsure whether your qualifications or work experience meet a school's criteria, contact the admissions team directly. Most are happy to confirm eligibility or clarify what they expect.

Once academic screening is complete, selectors review the personal statement and academic reference to understand each applicant's motivation, insight and suitability for the veterinary profession. Because most applicants will have strong predicted grades, your ability to demonstrate reflection, resilience and a realistic understanding of the career often makes the difference.

Your school or college reference supports this by providing evidence of your academic strengths, work ethic and character.

At this stage, admissions tutors make interview decisions based solely on the information in your UCAS form, so every detail matters. If your application doesn't meet either the academic or non-academic criteria, it cannot progress to interview and therefore cannot result in an offer.

The UCAS application form

All applications for UK veterinary medicine courses are submitted online through UCAS (the Universities and Colleges Admissions Service). The process is managed via your UCAS Hub account, which is both your application portal and your main source of guidance and updates.

The Hub allows you to:

- explore different university and course options;
- save favourite courses and track your progress;
- access advice on personal statements, interviews and student finance;
- complete and submit your UCAS application.

5| The UCAS Application

Most students register through their school or college using a buzzword provided by their tutor. Independent applicants can register directly.

Once logged in, you'll be asked for your year of entry, level of study, country of residence and subject interests. These details help UCAS tailor the guidance displayed in your Hub dashboard.

The application sections

Your UCAS application is divided into several parts.

1. **Personal information**

You will need to provide your name, contact details, nationality, residential status and fee information. You can also disclose any support needs or extenuating circumstances, for example, a disability, long-term illness, caring responsibilities or disruption to education.

2. **Education**

List all of your qualifications, both completed and pending. Include GCSEs (or equivalents), A levels, BTECs or Access to HE Diplomas. Accuracy is vital – ensure that exam boards, grades and dates are correct, as universities use this information to confirm eligibility for their courses.

3. **Employment and experience**

Here you can record details of any paid work or formal voluntary positions. Short-term placements, such as animal handling or veterinary shadowing, can instead be reflected upon in your personal statement.

4. **Course choices**

You may apply to a maximum of five courses. For veterinary medicine, however, you may only apply to four veterinary schools. The fifth choice can be used for a related subject (for example, bioveterinary science or zoology), or it can be left blank. If you are applying for deferred entry, you can indicate this here.

5. **Personal statement (new format from 2026 entry)**

From 2026 entry, UCAS replaced the single free-form personal statement with three structured questions, each with its own word or character limit (up to 4,000 characters in total).

These are designed to help you reflect more clearly on your motivation and preparation for the course.

You are asked to respond to three core themes:

- Motivation for the course – why do you want to study veterinary medicine?
- Preparation and suitability – how have your studies and experiences prepared you for the course?
- Exploration and experience – what have you done outside the classroom to develop your understanding of the profession?

This new format removes much of the stress of writing a single essay and encourages focused, reflective responses. You should still draw on your work experience, voluntary placements, independent learning and wider interests, showing what you have learnt and how this has shaped your motivation to become a vet.

6. **Reference (new format from 2026 entry)**

The reference section has also been simplified. From the 2026 entry, teachers or referees must answer a series of structured questions rather than providing a single free-form reference letter. They comment on:

- your academic readiness for university study;
- your attitude and approach to learning;
- any contextual information (such as mitigating circumstances or educational disadvantage).

If you are applying through your school or college, your application will first be sent to them for review and the reference will be added before submission. If you are applying independently, UCAS will contact your nominated referee directly to upload their response.

Final checks before submitting

Before submitting your UCAS application, make sure to:

- read the instructions carefully for each section;
- double-check all details (dates, grades, qualification titles and contact information);
- proofread for spelling and grammar errors;
- ask a teacher or adviser to review your application before it is sent.

Once your application is submitted, you can track its progress through UCAS Hub, from acknowledgement of receipt to interview invitations and final decisions.

Additional forms and questionnaires

Some veterinary schools request extra information after the UCAS deadline.

- Cambridge applicants must complete the My Cambridge Application by 22 October.
- Other universities, such as Bristol, RVC and Edinburgh, use supplementary questionnaires to collect details about work experience, motivation or understanding of the profession.

These forms are usually released shortly after the UCAS deadline, so check your email and UCAS Hub regularly.

> **Application timeline summary**
>
> **June–September:** Begin drafting your responses and finalise course choices
>
> **15 October:** UCAS submission deadline for veterinary medicine
>
> **October–January:** Complete supplementary forms and prepare for interviews
>
> **November–March:** Interview period
>
> **January–May:** Offers and decisions released via UCAS Hub

Submitting your application

When you've reviewed every section of your application and are confident that it's complete and accurate, you're ready to submit it through UCAS Hub.

If you are applying through your school or college, your application will first be sent to your referee for approval and submission. If you are applying independently, UCAS will contact your referee directly to upload their response before you can send it.

Before submitting, you will be asked to confirm that:

- all the information you've provided is accurate, complete and written in your own words;
- you understand that your application will be shared with all your chosen universities;
- you agree to abide by UCAS's terms and conditions.

Finally, you'll need to pay the UCAS application fee (for 2026 entry, this is £28.95 for up to five choices) to complete your submission.

Once you've submitted your application, you'll receive a confirmation email and can track its progress through UCAS Hub.

The reference

Once your application is complete, it will be sent to your referee for review and completion. This is usually someone who knows your academic performance well – typically your head of sixth form, personal tutor or subject teacher.

From 2026 entry, UCAS replaced the traditional free-form reference with a structured format. Instead of writing a long paragraph, referees now respond to a series of short sections that help universities assess your readiness for higher education.

Your referee will be asked to comment on three key areas:

- **Academic readiness**: how well you are prepared for the academic demands of university study.
- **Attitude and engagement**: your motivation, curiosity, resilience and contribution to the learning environment.
- **Contextual information**: any circumstances that may have affected your education or exam results, such as illness, caring responsibilities or other personal challenges.

Although the structure has changed, the purpose remains the same: to give admissions tutors an independent, evidence-based assessment of your strengths, potential and suitability for the course.

A strong reference will confirm your:

- consistent academic performance and predicted grades;
- enthusiasm for veterinary medicine;
- ability to work independently and collaboratively;
- personal qualities such as empathy, professionalism and perseverance.

Making a good impression

Your referee can only comment on what they've seen from you, so make sure you build a positive reputation long before you apply.

Get involved in your school or college community, show enthusiasm for your subjects and demonstrate curiosity beyond the curriculum, especially in biology and chemistry. Simple things like meeting deadlines, engaging in class discussions and offering to help at open evenings or school events all build evidence for a strong reference.

If you feel you haven't yet shown these qualities, don't panic – it's never too late to start. Begin now by:

- taking on new responsibilities or volunteering roles;
- talking openly with your teachers about your goals;
- showing steady improvement in your studies.

Predicted grades

As part of your reference, your referee will also predict your A level grades. Veterinary medicine is extremely competitive, and the minimum typical offer remains AAA, with some schools occasionally including an A*.

If your predicted grades are below this level, discuss it early with your teachers. You may be able to improve predictions by showing consistent progress or providing evidence of strong coursework and test results.

If your grades are significantly below the standard offer, you could:

- work more strategically and seek extra support in weaker areas.
- consider deferring your application to allow for an academic boost.
- contact admissions teams directly to ask about contextual or Gateway routes.

> **TIP!**
>
> Your reference and personal statement should complement each other. Where your personal statement shows your motivation and insight into the profession, your reference should reinforce that you have the discipline, maturity and work ethic to succeed once you get there.

What happens next?

Once you submit your UCAS application, you will receive an email confirmation from UCAS within a few hours. This confirms that your application has been received and sent to your chosen universities. You can then track your progress at any time through your UCAS Hub account, using the same login details you used to apply.

As soon as your application has been processed, your chosen veterinary schools will be able to view it. They cannot see where else you've applied, so you don't need to worry about your other course choices influencing their decision.

Most universities will send a short acknowledgement email confirming that they have received your application. Some may also provide instructions about next steps, for example, how to access their applicant portal, or when to expect communication about interviews or additional forms. Don't worry if you don't receive an acknowledgement straight away; not all veterinary schools send them.

From this point forward, check your emails and UCAS Hub regularly. Veterinary schools may contact you to:

- request supplementary information or questionnaires (e.g. Bristol's or RVC's work experience forms);
- invite you to attend an interview or selection day;
- update you on the progress of your application.

> **TIP!**
>
> Always check your junk or spam folder – university emails sometimes get filtered automatically. To avoid missing anything, add UCAS and your chosen universities to your email contacts list.

Once universities have made decisions, you'll see their responses in the 'Your Choices' section of UCAS Hub. This will show whether you've been invited to interview, received an offer or been unsuccessful.

Hearing back from veterinary schools

Veterinary schools receive a very high number of applications, so it can take time before you hear anything further. Most interviews take place between November and March, depending on the university's admissions timetable.

If you are shortlisted for interview, the invitation will usually arrive by email (occasionally via the university's applicant portal), and details will also appear in your UCAS Hub. Invitations typically include:

- the date and time of your interview or selection day;
- the format (online or in-person);
- any pre-reading or preparation tasks;
- information about what to bring with you.

If you haven't heard anything by late February, don't panic – many universities make decisions at different times. However, it's sensible to check your UCAS Hub and email folders regularly and to confirm that your contact details are up to date.

After interviews are complete, most universities aim to release decisions by March or April, in line with UCAS deadlines. Once you have received all your offers, you can make your firm and insurance choices through UCAS Hub before the stated decision deadline.

Other supporting documentation

Because work experience is such a vital part of the selection process, veterinary schools will often ask you to provide further details about your placements after you apply. This helps admissions tutors understand what you learnt, the range of experiences you gained and how these have influenced your motivation to study veterinary medicine.

Most veterinary schools now use online questionnaires or reflective forms rather than contacting placements directly. Examples include:

- the RVC Work Experience Questionnaire;
- the Bristol Supplementary Assessment Questionnaire;
- the Edinburgh Work Experience Summary (WES) Form.

These forms are usually sent to applicants shortly after the 15 October UCAS deadline, and you'll be given a few weeks to complete them. They often ask you to describe:

- the types of placements you've undertaken (e.g. small animal, farm, equine, laboratory, etc.);
- what you observed and learnt;
- examples of your teamwork, communication or problem solving;
- how your experiences have confirmed your commitment to becoming a vet.

While universities rarely contact placement providers directly, they may request references or confirmation if needed; for example, the RVC occasionally asks for contact details to verify experience.

It's therefore a good idea to keep in touch with your supervisors and to ask for a short reference letter or written confirmation at the end of each placement, outlining what you did and how you performed. This will make it easier if a university later asks for evidence.

When requesting a reference, politely ask your placement provider to include:

- your dates of placement;
- a brief description of your responsibilities;
- a short comment on your reliability, professionalism and attitude.

Remember that every interaction counts. Admissions tutors value comments from people who can genuinely say you were enthusiastic, thoughtful and a pleasure to have around – qualities that are just as important as academic achievement in this profession.

Admissions tests

For 2026 entry, the only veterinary school in the UK that requires an admissions test is the University of Cambridge. All other vet schools make their selection based on academic achievement, work experience and interview performance, and there is no longer any requirement to sit the UCAT or BMAT.

Cambridge applicants must take the Engineering and Science Admissions Test (ESAT), introduced to replace the previous Natural Sciences Admissions Assessment (NSAA). The ESAT assesses problem-solving ability and scientific understanding in mathematics, biology, chemistry and physics.

Applicants for Veterinary Medicine are required to sit three 40-minute multiple-choice papers, including:

- mathematics 1 (compulsory for all candidates);
- biology;
- chemistry.

The ESAT is computer-based and is taken at Pearson VUE test centres in mid-October (for 2026 entry, the test dates were 9 and 10 October 2025). It can only be taken once per application cycle.

Scores are based on the total number of correct answers (no negative marking). Cambridge colleges use these results alongside A level or equivalent performance, the UCAS application and the interview when deciding whom to offer places to.

Full details, including registration deadlines, fees, bursary schemes and free preparation materials, are available on the University of Cambridge Undergraduate Study website.

UCAS Extra

If you've used all four of your veterinary medicine choices and don't receive any offers, or if you change your mind about where or what you'd like to study, you may be eligible to use UCAS Extra.

UCAS Extra is a free service that allows applicants one application at a time to courses that still have available places. It runs from the end of February until early July and is accessed directly through your UCAS Hub account.

You can apply to one course at a time, wait for a decision, and if you are unsuccessful, choose another. This continues until you either receive an offer or the Extra period ends.

To use UCAS Extra, you must have:

- used all five UCAS choices;
- received no offers, or declined any you received.

If you already hold an offer, you'll need to decline it before using Extra, so only do this if you're absolutely sure.

It's important to note that veterinary medicine rarely appears in UCAS Extra, as courses are usually full after the initial application round. However, it's always worth checking, as places can occasionally become available. Even if not, you may find related courses, such as bioveterinary science, animal science or zoology, which can be useful alternative routes if you plan to reapply later.

What to do if you are rejected

If you're unsuccessful and receive rejections from one or more of your veterinary school choices, don't panic – this is a common outcome in such a competitive field. Remember that thousands of applicants apply for a limited number of places each year, so rejections often reflect intense competition rather than a lack of ability.

If you receive four rejections, take time to reflect on your application and identify what you could improve for next time. You can:

- **Contact admissions departments** to politely request feedback. Many veterinary schools will offer brief guidance on why your application wasn't successful – this could relate to academic requirements, work experience or interview performance.
- **Evaluate your academic profile**: if your predicted or achieved grades were below the standard offer, focus on improving them before reapplying.
- **Build your experience further**: try to gain additional placements, especially in areas you haven't covered yet (e.g. mixed practice, farm, equine).
- **Refine your personal statement** using the feedback you receive and by reflecting on what you've learnt from your experiences.

If you meet the entry requirements but do not hold an offer after results day, you can explore UCAS Clearing. Veterinary schools rarely have spaces available, but it's always worth checking the UCAS course search tool in August. Occasionally, places become available due to applicants withdrawing or missing their grades.

If you do contact a veterinary school about potential Clearing places, make sure you have:

- your UCAS ID and grades ready;
- your personal statement and reference accessible in case they ask about your experience or motivation.

Be prepared for the possibility of a short-notice interview, as veterinary schools will still want to assess your suitability.

If you're still determined to pursue a career in veterinary medicine, consider taking a gap year to gain more experience, improve your academic results or strengthen your application. Many successful applicants are reapplicants who used this time effectively.

Deferring entry and taking a gap year

The UCAS system allows you to apply for veterinary medicine while still in Year 13, but to request deferred entry, meaning you would begin your studies the following academic year. In this case, you must still meet all offer conditions (such as your A level grades) in the year of application.

Most veterinary schools are supportive of deferred entry, provided you have a constructive plan for your year out. Common reasons include:

- gaining additional work experience in animal care, farms or veterinary practices;
- travelling or volunteering abroad in animal-related projects;
- taking up employment to develop your communication, teamwork or resilience;
- studying or completing short courses to strengthen your academic background.

Of these, gaining more hands-on experience is the reason most likely to be viewed favourably by veterinary schools. A well-planned gap year can demonstrate motivation, maturity and commitment to the profession, especially if your first round of applications was unsuccessful or your work experience was limited.

Alternatively, you may choose to wait until after receiving your A level results to apply during your gap year. This approach allows you to submit a stronger, more confident application once your academic results and additional experience are confirmed.

If you are planning to defer or apply post-qualification, make sure you can clearly explain your gap year plans in your application or interview. Many veterinary schools will ask how your time away from study will contribute to your personal and professional growth.

Transferring from another degree

If you are certain that you want to become a veterinary surgeon, it is not advisable to start a different degree with the intention of transferring partway through. Although this might seem like a shortcut, direct transfers into veterinary medicine are not possible at UK veterinary schools.

This is because the veterinary curriculum includes core, specialist subjects, such as veterinary anatomy, physiology and animal husbandry, that are taught from the very beginning of the degree. These modules are essential to later clinical training and cannot be skipped or replaced with credits from another course.

In addition, veterinary schools operate with limited cohort sizes and rarely have spare places available mid-programme, meaning that even if you have completed a related course, you would still need to start again from Year 1.

If you are interested in becoming a vet but have already started or completed a different degree, a more realistic option is to apply as a graduate entrant. Some universities offer graduate entry or accelerated veterinary medicine programmes, while others consider graduates for standard five-year courses. This route allows you to use your first degree as a foundation, demonstrating academic maturity and commitment to the profession.

For more on graduate entry and the benefits of this pathway, see Chapter 4.

Case study

After underperforming in her GCSEs, Georgia started her A levels in non-science subjects as she was told there was no way she could pursue her dream of becoming a vet. After completing her AS exams in these subjects, she changed schools, retook her GCSEs and commenced a new A level programme. Things may not have gone to plan for Georgia, but she has graduated from the world's leading veterinary school, the Royal Veterinary College, with a BSc in Bioveterinary Science and commenced her studies on their veterinary science programme. It's not the route she wanted to take, but when life threw her a series of curveballs, she went along for the ride! Here, Georgia reflects on her journey to vet school and the trials and tribulations that she has encountered along the way. Georgia's story is one of great perseverance and resilience, and shows that with determination and focus, you can always succeed.

'My journey to veterinary medicine has been anything but "easy". As with most vet school applicants, I have wanted to become a vet for as long as I can remember. From the moment I began my first work experience placement at the age of 15, I knew this would be my dream job and I would do anything to achieve it.

'The struggles I have faced on this journey, including getting the grades, UCAS applications, interviews and, of course, a global pandemic, have been some of the most difficult challenges of my academic life. If there has been anything that I have learnt from the past six years, it is that perseverance really does pay off and if you want something enough, it will happen!

'I transferred to MPW college from my existing secondary school as not achieving the GCSE grades I had hoped for meant I couldn't study science at A level standard. So, I decided to leave that school, move into the city and get to work. I worked hard for three years, lived away from my family for most of the academic year and consumed myself in my GCSE and then A level studies. I managed to secure an offer from RVC, my dream university, as well as two others. I was overjoyed! This was going to be my moment. When it finally came to me receiving my A level grades, you can imagine the shock of finding out I had narrowly missed out on the grades I needed for my offer. So … what now?

'After all of that hard work and accumulating 28 weeks' worth experience to not get a place at vet school, I would be lying if I said I didn't feel like giving up at that moment. My options were to leave everything I had worked towards right there or take up the offer of Bioveterinary Science at RVC, which I could use as a platform to apply for Veterinary Medicine as a graduate. Ultimately, the three-year course at my dream university was a no-brainer and I had to at least try.

'Choosing to move to a solely veterinary-orientated university when you are not studying that degree, and it's your lifelong passion, didn't feel like my smartest choice – it was difficult to be surrounded by what could have been. Studying an academically rigorous undergraduate degree that is not your first choice can be incredibly hard at times, and it can be tough to motivate yourself to keep going.

'There were definitely times when I thought I wouldn't be able to get through it, but immersing myself into university life really helped. I made some really great friends, which made the situation a lot easier. It was great to be able to talk to them (as well as my tutors and my family) about how I was feeling when things were tough – I quickly realised that many people felt the same way as I did and I wasn't on my own. I took part in many social events and joined sports teams and societies. Throwing myself into things taught me to appreciate the experience of university as a whole in my own development.

'My journey to veterinary school may not have been a smooth ride, but looking back on my decisions now, I am really happy with how everything turned out. There are so many benefits of studying for an undergraduate degree before pursuing veterinary medicine that are often overlooked. Some of these benefits are that you are able to get used to the university's way of running things, such as exams, in advance, as well as developing better study habits more aligned with the demands of higher level study. I met some amazing people, including tutors, who led me into avenues of study that I wouldn't have considered otherwise and found that I really enjoyed. In addition, when you come to apply again in the future, you will have an additional three years' worth of experience to talk about, which is always a plus!

'Preparing to apply again for veterinary medicine can be really daunting. You are filled with anxiety about missing out again, and you may worry that you are too old, but in all honesty, none of that matters in the slightest. Make sure you are well prepared and have a good range of work experience to talk about, and the rest will fall into place.

'My top tips for applying to veterinary medicine as a graduate are:

1. **Work experience**: this can be really difficult to get while studying a full-time degree. You normally have 18 months prior to submitting your application to undertake the required amount of work experience. You really want to avoid doing this in your final degree year as you will have very little time, so I recommend at the end of your second year really cramming in as much as you can, and maybe go lambing for a few weeks over Easter if it's possible around exams.
2. **Hobbies**: one thing I learnt from my endless experience with veterinary medicine applications is that they really want to know who you are and what you enjoy outside of the scientific community. It's great that you wrote a 35-page research article on the effects of Bovine Viral Diarrhoea Virus on the expression of genes associated with pregnancy recognition in cattle, but they want to see who YOU are! Take up painting, go rock climbing – the world is your oyster!
3. **University life**: this point is an extension from the last, try and get involved in university clubs and social events as much as possible. Get to know the lecturers and become an active member of the university. It helps to show on your application that you have really taken advantage of being an undergraduate student and why they should want you to contribute to their university!

'My one final piece of advice for any Bioveterinary Science undergraduate that wants to become a vet is that this degree is just a stepping stone to get you to where you want to be. It's not forever, and it doesn't mean you will be any less of an amazing vet! If anything, it will make you a lot more competent than most of the first-time degree vets, believe me! Applying to postgraduate veterinary medicine is another challenge in itself, but it's not impossible. The only thing you need is belief in yourself and a lot of determination. Work hard and you will reap the benefits!'

Fact: Young goats pick up accents from one another.

6 | No one likes a copycat
The personal statement

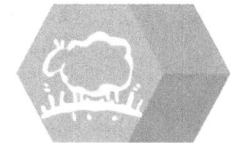

One of the most important parts of your application is the section where you explain why you want to study veterinary medicine and show your understanding of the profession. This is where admissions tutors assess not just your academic potential, but your motivation, commitment and suitability for the veterinary profession.

Until recently, applicants wrote a single 4,000-character personal statement. However, from 2026 entry onwards, UCAS has replaced this with three structured questions. This new approach is designed to make the process fairer, more focused and easier for universities to compare applicants.

The three UCAS questions are:

1. **Motivation for the course**: why do you want to study this course?
2. **Preparation for the course through learning**: how have your studies so far helped you to prepare?
3. **Preparation through experience**: what have you done outside of formal education to explore and prepare for the course?

Each question has a maximum word limit rather than a shared character count (currently set at around 1,000 words total, divided across the three responses).

Each question has its own text box, but the total combined limit remains 4,000 characters (including spaces), which you can divide between the three answers as you wish.

What admissions tutors are looking for

Regardless of the different format, admissions tutors still want to see:

- **Motivation**: a clear, well-reasoned explanation of why you want to be a vet and what has inspired this decision.
- **Exploration**: genuine engagement with the profession through relevant work experience, volunteering or research.

- **Suitability**: the personal attributes, such as empathy, communication skills, resilience and teamwork, that demonstrate you will thrive in a demanding course and career.

When comparing academically strong candidates, this section often becomes the deciding factor for who is invited to interview. A response that lacks reflection or structure, or that is overly descriptive, may put you at a disadvantage.

Sections of the personal statement

The new UCAS format breaks your written section into three structured questions. These still cover the same themes as a traditional personal statement, but they encourage more focused and reflective answers.

Below is guidance on how to approach each section, with examples of what veterinary schools will expect.

1. **Motivation for the course**: why do you want to study this course or subject?

Admissions tutors want to understand why you want to become a vet and, crucially, that your interest is genuine and informed. Avoid opening with overused phrases like 'I've always wanted to be a vet because I love animals and science'. This tells them little about you as an individual.

Instead, describe what sparked your interest and how it has grown. This might include:

- a formative experience, such as observing a vet during work experience or caring for your own animals;
- a moment that inspired curiosity about animal health, behaviour or biology;
- an aspect of science or problem solving that you find rewarding and that links naturally to veterinary medicine.

Admissions tutors are not looking for dramatic stories – they want honest insight. Keep your explanation personal, specific and clearly linked to what you've since done to explore the profession further.

> **TIP!**
>
> Don't waste words explaining what veterinary medicine is – they already know. Focus instead on why it matters to you.

2. **Preparedness for the course through learning**: how have your qualifications and studies helped you to prepare for this course or subject?

This question allows you to show how your studies and intellectual interests have prepared you for the demands of a veterinary degree.

Highlight examples from school or independent study that demonstrate curiosity, persistence and scientific thinking. For example:

- topics in biology, chemistry or animal physiology that captured your interest;
- practical or investigative work where you developed observation, data handling or analytical skills;
- wider reading, podcasts or journal articles that deepened your understanding of issues such as animal welfare, disease control or sustainability.

Show that you can make connections between what you've learnt and the real-world challenges of veterinary practice. Avoid vague phrases like 'I enjoy biology' – instead, explain what you found fascinating and why.

If you've undertaken an Extended Project Qualification (EPQ) or similar research, summarise what you learnt and how it reinforced your decision to pursue this course.

3. **Preparation through other experiences**: what else have you done to prepare outside of education, and why are these experiences useful?

This is where you demonstrate that you've gained a realistic understanding of the veterinary profession through hands-on or virtual experiences.

Discuss your work experience first. Be clear about where you went, what you observed and, most importantly, what you learnt. Rather than listing placements, reflect on key takeaways, such as:

- the importance of teamwork and communication within a veterinary practice;
- balancing clinical care with compassion for clients;
- the emotional and physical demands of animal work.

You can also include voluntary work (e.g. animal shelters, farms, stables, wildlife centres) and non-clinical roles that developed transferable skills like leadership, organisation or resilience.

If your access to placements was limited, explain how you broadened your understanding in other ways, such as completing Nottingham's Virtual Work Experience course, following RCVS or BVA updates or learning through documentaries and podcasts. What matters most is reflection, not the number of hours.

Throughout your answers, you should also evidence key personal qualities sought by veterinary schools:

- communication and empathy;
- teamwork and reliability;
- manual dexterity and practical awareness;
- resilience, organisation and attention to detail.

You can draw on examples from school, part-time work, sport or other achievements – anything that illustrates the qualities required of a good vet.

> **TIP!**
>
> Aim to show variety and commitment. Depth of reflection counts for more than the number of placements listed.

Summary: planning your responses

If you're unsure what to include in your UCAS answers, start by jotting down ideas under the three new question areas. These prompts will help you identify the most relevant experiences and reflections to include.

1. **Why do you want to study this course or subject?**
   - What first sparked your interest in veterinary medicine?
   - Have any particular experiences, books or encounters strengthened that interest?
   - What aspects of veterinary work appeal to you most – problem solving, science, working with people or caring for animals?
   - Can you link your motivation to specific examples from your experiences or studies?
2. **How have your qualifications and studies helped you to prepare for this course or subject?**
   - Which topics from your A levels or other studies have been most relevant or inspiring?
   - Have you completed any research projects, EPQs or coursework related to animal science, biology or chemistry?
   - What skills have you developed through your studies that will help you succeed on a veterinary degree (e.g. analysis, attention to detail, practical skills)?
   - How have your academic interests evolved as you've learnt more about science and animal health?

3. **What else have you done to prepare outside of education, and why are these experiences useful?**
    - What veterinary or animal-related placements have you completed, and what did you learn from them?
    - Have you observed any interesting cases or developed key insights about communication, teamwork or animal care?
    - How have you worked with others – vets, nurses, clients or peers – and what did you learn from these interactions?
    - Do you have achievements, positions of responsibility or activities (sport, music, volunteering) that demonstrate your dedication, leadership or teamwork skills?
    - What skills or qualities have you gained from these experiences that would help you thrive at veterinary school and as a future vet?

> **TIP!**
>
> Once you've answered these questions in note form, review your responses for common themes. These will form the backbone of your final UCAS answers, helping you write with focus, depth and authenticity.

Using Artificial Intelligence (AI) in your UCAS application

Artificial Intelligence (AI) tools such as ChatGPT, Grammarly or other writing assistants are increasingly common in education, and it's understandable that applicants may wonder whether they can use them to help prepare their UCAS responses. However, when it comes to your veterinary medicine application, it's vital to understand what is and isn't allowed.

Your declaration to UCAS

When you submit your UCAS application, you must confirm that your written responses are entirely your own work. This includes the new question-based personal statement format. UCAS explicitly states that using AI to write or heavily edit your responses counts as presenting work that isn't your own, and could lead to your application being withdrawn.

Universities and UCAS use similarity detection tools to flag copied or formulaic text. If large sections of your answers appear AI-generated or identical to other submissions, it may raise concerns about authenticity. Admissions tutors are highly experienced at spotting generic or impersonal writing, especially in vocational subjects such as veterinary medicine, where reflection and individuality are key.

Why overusing AI can harm your application

Even if not detected formally, heavy use of AI can still work against you. AI-generated writing often:

- sounds polished but lacks personality or insight;
- includes generic reflections that could apply to any applicant ('I am passionate about science and helping animals');
- misses specific details about your experiences, such as placements, challenges or moments of learning;
- uses language or phrasing that doesn't match the style of a sixth-form student.

Admissions tutors want to get a sense of you – your motivation, thought process and communication skills. An over-edited or artificially perfect response can make it harder for them to see that.

How you can use AI safely

AI can still be a useful support tool if used responsibly. The key is to ensure that your final responses are entirely written in your own words. You might use AI to:

- Brainstorm ideas for what to include (e.g. 'What kinds of experiences might a vet applicant reflect on?').
- Check your spelling, grammar or sentence clarity.
- Suggest ways to improve flow or reduce repetition.
- Generate questions to help you think more deeply about your experiences ('What did this placement teach me about teamwork or animal welfare?').

However, the writing and reflection must always come from you. Use AI as a thinking partner, not a ghostwriter.

Summary

Using AI to brainstorm or check your writing can help you feel more confident, but using it to write your UCAS answers for you can have serious consequences. Remember:

- Your UCAS responses must be your own independent work.
- AI-written content can make your application sound impersonal and generic.
- Admissions tutors value honesty, reflection and individuality far more than perfect phrasing.

Things to avoid

Writing your UCAS answers for veterinary medicine can take time, and that's completely normal. The key is to produce something authentic, thoughtful and relevant. Here are some common pitfalls to avoid.

1. **Writing too little**

UCAS allows up to 4,000 characters across your three responses, and you should aim to use as much of that space as possible. A short or underdeveloped response suggests a lack of reflection or motivation. Make every word count by giving clear examples, explaining what you learnt, and linking your experiences directly to veterinary medicine.

2. **Listing without reflecting**

Simply describing what you did – 'I shadowed a vet', 'I volunteered at a shelter' – is not enough. You must reflect on what you learnt, how it developed your skills and how it strengthened your motivation. Admissions tutors are looking for depth, not just activity.

3. **Forgetting to make it personal**

The most memorable statements sound genuine. Use your own experiences and observations – what surprised you, challenged you or inspired you. Avoid generic phrases that could belong to anyone.

4. **Sounding negative**

Keep your tone positive. You don't need to mention aspects of the course or career that you might find off-putting. Focus on what attracts you and how you've prepared to meet the challenges of veterinary study.

5. **Explaining the obvious**

You don't need to lecture admissions tutors about what veterinary surgeons do or what the course involves – they already know. Use your space to discuss your understanding of the profession and what draws you to it.

6. **Mentioning money or prestige**

Avoid talking about salary, job security or social status. Admissions tutors want to see a genuine commitment to animal health and welfare, not financial motivation.

7. **Using clichés and stock phrases**

Phrases such as 'I have always loved animals' or 'I've wanted to be a vet since I was a child' are overused. If these ideas are true for you, express them in a way that's specific and personal, for example, by referring to a real experience that brought your interest to life.

8. **Losing focus**

Your responses should centre on veterinary medicine. If your most passionate writing is about unrelated subjects, refocus it to highlight how your interests connect to science, problem solving or animal care.

9. **Overcomplicating your language**

Clear, precise writing always reads better than overly elaborate phrasing. Avoid using a thesaurus for every sentence – it's more important that your responses sound natural and confident.

10. **Using Artificial Intelligence (AI)**

UCAS now requires applicants to confirm that their responses are entirely their own work. Using AI tools such as ChatGPT or AI writing assistants to generate or edit your UCAS responses is not permitted and could result in your application being withdrawn.

You can, however, use AI ethically for planning or research, for instance, to brainstorm topics or find reliable sources, as long as the final writing is your own.

Example personal statements

The example responses below show how an applicant might structure their written answers for veterinary medicine.

There is no single perfect way to write a UCAS response, as every applicant's experiences and motivations are different. What matters is that your writing feels authentic, reflective and personal.

There are no right or wrong answers – only ways to express your journey in a genuine and thoughtful way. As long as your writing is personal and meaningful to you, you will have achieved your goal.

> **Remember:** be concise and authentic. This doesn't mean you have to be outgoing or try to sound impressive – it means you should make your writing honest and true to who you are.
>
> Relate everything back to yourself:
>
> - What skills and qualities can you bring to the course?
> - How have you developed these over time, both inside and outside the classroom?

6| The Personal Statement

> Your individuality comes from how you reflect on your experiences. While many applicants will have similar work experience, no one will have your combination of insights, challenges and growth. Think carefully about what makes your perspective unique and what you most want the university to understand about you, then communicate that clearly and confidently.

Example personal statement 1

1. Why do you want to study veterinary medicine?

Standing knee-deep in mud, desperately trying to prevent an embryo from defrosting as the local vet manoeuvred a heifer into the crush, is perhaps my most vivid memory of my placement in Ireland. Yet it was in that crucial moment – despite the torrential rain and the angry cows – that I realised that the prospect of a career in veterinary medicine provided enough drive to overcome the significant hurdles that pursuing it would present.

Since then, I have explored all aspects of the profession, from the highs of bringing new life into the world during lambing season to the lows of euthanasia within a small practice. What draws me most to veterinary medicine is the balance between intellectual challenge, practical skill and the privilege of working for both animals and their owners. The profession's blend of science, empathy and lifelong learning continues to inspire me.

2. How have your learning and studies prepared you for the course?

By studying biology, I have developed a strong understanding of physiology, from the basis of movement through antagonistic muscle action to resistance against infection by the immune system. In practice, I have witnessed the importance of having a strong scientific knowledge in order to recognise symptoms and act accordingly in terms of diagnostics and treatment.

Studying chemistry has enlightened me to the intricate nature of pharmacology, and how the precise structural formula of a drug is so important to the outcome of the patient. The development of my problem-solving skills through chemistry will also prove invaluable when facing the diagnostic puzzles of veterinary medicine. My analytical skills have grown significantly through English literature, which became useful when assisting a vet in diagnosing a complex case of canine pyometra, interpreting ultrasound scans and contributing to the final diagnosis.

My Extended Project Qualification on neurodegenerative diseases in ruminants allowed me to study a complex organ in depth and further increased my fascination with livestock diseases. Over the year, I also plan to complete an Artificial Insemination course to strengthen my livestock handling skills.

3. What else have you done to prepare, and how has this supported your interest?

In pursuit of a career in this field, I have gained experience across a wide range of placements, from working on a 22,000-sow unit to implanting over 100 CIDRs on a cattle farm, and I remain in awe of the intricate complexity of animal biology. My weekly placement at my local practice has enabled me to develop practical skills such as bandaging, intubation and suturing, as well as to handle sensitive interactions with both patients and owners.

The future of veterinary medicine excites me; the possibilities of biomechanics and new developments in oncology that I witnessed while attending specialist lectures at congress were particularly fascinating. More recently, I volunteered at a wildlife sanctuary in Australia, working alongside native fauna and researching Koala Retrovirus. This enabled me to explore potential treatment concepts such as nanomedicine to improve outcomes for koalas with compromised immune systems.

Outside of placements, I have been running a blog on my university application since 2015, accredited by organisations such as Veterinary Times, and my articles have been featured both online and in my college magazine. As an author and editor for the *Young Scientist Journal*, I published an article on the use of Tyrosine Kinase Inhibitors in veterinary chemotherapy. Attending events such as VetFest and VetsSouth has expanded my knowledge and allowed me to converse with leading veterinarians.

My unwavering passion for the field, combined with my enthusiasm for research, dedication to animal welfare and practical experience to date, have consolidated my belief that veterinary medicine is the perfect career choice for me.

Example personal statement 2

1. Why do you want to study veterinary medicine?

My passion for animal care began long before I understood veterinary medicine as a profession. Growing up, our home felt like a small rehabilitation centre, where I helped my parents treat sick and injured stray animals. What I once assumed was normal gradually became the foundation of a lifelong aspiration. When I was old enough to recognise that I wanted to become a vet, I began seeking placements, internships and courses, each one strengthening my motivation and confirming my commitment to the profession.

Living across Turkey, China, South Africa and Sweden has shown me that although veterinary practice differs between cultures, the core principles of welfare, regulation and patient care remain universal. Seeing this global perspective reinforced my desire to join a profession that combines science, compassion and service. My blog documents my experiences across veterinary surgeries, university anatomy classes, ranches, farms, a cattery and wildlife reserves, reflecting both the variety and the depth of my engagement with the field.

2. How have your learning and studies prepared you for the course?

Through extensive placements across Turkey, the UK and China, including six months in an international pet hospital, I have observed consultations, joined clinical case discussions and assisted in surgeries such as castrations, ovariohysterectomies, amputations and mass removals. Observing vets interpret diagnostic tests taught me the importance of chemistry in prescribing safely, while work in a cattery highlighted the value of empathy and clear communication. These experiences encouraged me to study A level psychology to better understand behaviour, welfare and the science of human–animal interactions.

The Vetsim and VetMedic courses at Nottingham University further developed my scientific interest. Practical sessions, conferences and a genetic engineering workshop deepened my appreciation for the research that underpins veterinary decision-making. My internship at Ankara University's research farm strengthened my understanding of anatomy and physiology, as I handled cattle and sheep daily and participated in laboratory sessions working on cadavers' digestive and respiratory systems. These experiences reinforced why subjects such as biology and chemistry are essential foundations for veterinary study.

My academic journey has therefore equipped me with analytical skills, resilience and a genuine curiosity about the biological sciences that underpin clinical practice.

3. What else have you done to prepare, and how has this supported your interest?

Working with wild animals at an African game reserve offered a powerful insight into the emotional complexity of veterinary work. Helping a hyena recover contrasted sharply with the sadness of euthanising young puppies due to financial constraints, and even using one as a cadaver for teaching. This experience highlighted the differences between shelter and private practice and taught me to balance compassion with professional responsibility.

Beyond clinical work, I have organised community projects such as rescuing newborn sea turtles, teaching me how meaningful a single intervention can be for wider ecology. As a show jumper who has ridden since the age of four, I have learnt discipline, resilience and responsibility. Owning horses and shadowing stable vets taught me basic equine care, emergency management and the importance of preventative medicine. Achieving second place in show jumping at the Longines China Tour and receiving commendation from the Chamber of Commerce reflect my determination to excel.

Having lived and studied across several countries, I have become trilingual and developed strong cultural awareness, tolerance and empathy. I work well both independently and in teams, and I remain composed under pressure, qualities that will help me meet the demands of veterinary training. I look forward to contributing to clinical practice, public health work and research. For me, veterinary medicine is not just a career but a meaningful opportunity to support animals, their owners and the communities they belong to.

Example personal statement 3

1. Why do you want to study veterinary medicine?

Watching my first dog spay at 14, I was captivated by the precision, coordination and anatomical understanding required of the surgeon. Since then, I have actively sought to strengthen my understanding of the profession, immersing myself in more than 18 weeks of veterinary experience across small animal, farm, equine, mixed and international settings.

What motivates me most is the combination of scientific challenge, practical skill and the privilege of supporting both animals and their owners. Observing vets navigate complex clinical, ethical and financial decisions has shown me that veterinary medicine is a profession that demands compassion, resilience and adaptability. My experiences have continually reaffirmed that this dynamic and multifaceted career is the right path for me.

2. How have your learning and studies prepared you for the course?

My academic background has prepared me well for veterinary study. Key biology modules, such as parasitology and immunology, have allowed me to draw parallels between human and veterinary medicine, deepening my understanding of infectious disease and immune function. Statistical and bioinformatics modules have strengthened my analytical and problem-solving skills, helping me interpret data and work logically through scientific questions.

During placements, I was able to apply scientific principles directly. In small animal practice, understanding anatomy and physiology helped me appreciate clinical decision-making, particularly when observing terminal cases such as canine carcinoma. In Ghana, I assisted with preliminary checks, drew up medication and helped with surgical procedures, including closing a hernia repair using simple interrupted sutures. Limited resources often required creativity and problem solving, such as constructing a makeshift cast from masking tape and a sample tube for a kitten's suspected fracture.

Farm placements reinforced the link between veterinary medicine and public health. Observing dairy, poultry and lambing operations showed me how vets safeguard food quality and animal welfare while balancing practical and economic considerations. Equine placements enhanced my understanding of lameness diagnostics, metabolic disorders and reproductive management, while shadowing a neurectomy and assisting at a stud farm helped me appreciate the complexity of elite horse care.

3. What else have you done to prepare, and how has this supported your interest?

My wider experiences have strengthened my resilience, leadership and communication – qualities essential for veterinary medicine. Working at an equine stables as a riding instructor taught me to lead groups safely, explain technical concepts clearly and remain calm in unpredictable situations. Competing nationally in show jumping developed discipline, dedication and teamwork, while owning my own horses has given me confidence handling large animals and understanding preventative care.

Volunteering and charity work have shaped my empathy and commitment to community welfare. Completing my Duke of Edinburgh Gold Award and serving as a charity representative at school sparked a passion for service that led me to volunteer in Kenya for six weeks, where I taught a class of 20 pupils. On returning home, I raised £2,000 and initiated a 12-month renovation project, strengthening my organisation and perseverance.

At university, I have fundraised for Guide Dogs and earned my Level 1 My Guide certificate, supporting visually impaired individuals. As a STEM Ambassador, I visit disadvantaged schools to inspire young people in science, developing skills in explaining complex ideas clearly – an invaluable skill when communicating diagnoses to clients. I am also an active member of the biology, snowsports and art societies, and hope to volunteer with CommuniTea and as a zoology specimens volunteer.

My enthusiasm, self-motivation and intellectual curiosity, coupled with my practical experience, make me well suited to the veterinary profession. I look forward to beginning my training and to performing my first dog spay from the other side of the operating table.

General tips

Writing about yourself can be challenging, but keeping your responses authentic and focused will make a lasting impression. The following advice applies whether you are writing a traditional personal statement or completing the new UCAS questions.

- **Be authentic**: never copy someone else's writing. It won't reflect you, and plagiarism is taken very seriously by universities. The clue is in the name – it's personal.
- **Avoid using quotes**: admissions tutors want to hear your voice, not someone else's words.
- **Proofread carefully**: check for spelling or grammatical errors, ideally by printing a copy to review on paper.
- **Ask for feedback**: have one or two trusted people, such as a teacher or careers adviser, read your draft for clarity and flow. Avoid showing it to too many people, as opinions will vary and can make your writing less personal.
- **Keep a copy**: review what you've written before your interview, as selectors often ask you to expand on examples or ideas you've mentioned.
- **Reflect, don't list**: the best responses explain what you learnt from each experience, rather than simply describing what you did.
- **Highlight your development**: unique experiences are valuable when you show how they helped you grow as a person and confirmed your decision to study veterinary medicine.

> **Fact**: Horses use facial expressions to communicate with each other.

7 | So why did the chicken cross the road?
The interview

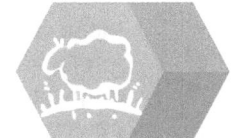

Once your written application has been submitted, the next stage is demonstrating your suitability in person. The interview is your opportunity to expand on the points you made in your UCAS responses and to show admissions tutors who you are beyond your application form.

If you meet the entry criteria and your application demonstrates the qualities veterinary schools are looking for, you may be invited to interview. This allows admissions tutors to assess whether the impression created by your written application is accurate and to evaluate your motivation, communication skills and potential to succeed on the course.

In this section, we'll look at the two main interview formats used by veterinary schools – the Multiple Mini Interview (MMI) and the panel interview – along with practical advice on preparation and general tips for success. Applicants may be invited to interview at any point between November and March, so it's important to start preparing as soon as your application has been submitted.

The purpose of the interview

Once you are invited to interview, you've already met the academic and work experience requirements, but selectors now want to learn more about you as a person. The interview is designed to assess your motivation, suitability and understanding of the veterinary profession.

Interviewers may explore areas such as:

- your attitude towards animal welfare and ethical issues;
- your awareness of the realities and demands of a veterinary career;
- your maturity, resilience and ability to manage stress;
- your capacity to cope with the pace and pressure of a long, demanding course.

They will already have access to your UCAS form, reference and any supporting statements from your work experience supervisors, so the interview allows them to test the picture those documents present.

Multiple Mini Interviews (MMIs)

Most veterinary schools now use the Multiple Mini Interview (MMI) format rather than traditional panel interviews. MMIs are designed to give a fairer, more rounded picture of each applicant's abilities and personal qualities.

Instead of a single interview, you move through a series of short stations, each focusing on a specific task or question. These might assess your communication skills, ethical reasoning, data interpretation or manual dexterity, as well as your ability to think logically and stay calm under pressure.

At each station, you'll be given written or verbal instructions explaining what to do. Listen and read carefully before responding. Remember that there are rarely 'right' or 'wrong' answers – interviewers are more interested in how you think, reason and communicate than in whether you reach a particular conclusion.

Vet schools have adopted MMIs for two main reasons:

1. Research shows they are a better predictor of future performance than traditional panel interviews.
2. They make it harder for candidates to rely on rehearsed answers, allowing interviewers to assess genuine communication and problem-solving skills.

Some universities keep the details of their MMI format confidential, while others provide sample questions or station outlines on their websites. Always read the interview invitation carefully and follow any pre-interview instructions provided.

Example MMI stations

Below are examples of the types of stations that may appear in a veterinary school MMI. The exact format will vary between universities, but these illustrate the range of skills and attributes typically assessed.

Practical skills and instruction-following
You may be asked to follow a set of written instructions – for example, using wire to construct a geometric shape with specified dimensions and angles. Tasks like this assess your ability to interpret information accurately, follow instructions precisely and demonstrate manual dexterity.

Numerical and drug calculations
A calculation station might involve determining a drug dosage based on the weight of an animal and adjusting the amount under different

conditions (e.g. reducing the dose by 40% for a particular health factor). These tasks test your confidence with basic maths, accuracy under pressure and understanding of proportional reasoning.

Communication and empathy
You could be asked to role-play a scenario such as breaking difficult news to an owner whose pet has died. Interviewers will look for empathy, professionalism and the ability to communicate clearly and sensitively without becoming overly emotional.

Ethical reasoning and animal welfare
A scenario might ask how you would respond if your dog found an injured wild animal, such as a badger. You would be expected to identify the animal welfare issues, discuss potential causes, outline what immediate action you would take and reference relevant organisations such as the RSPCA or local authorities.

Data interpretation
You may be given a graph or table – for instance, comparing animal growth rates and feed costs across different farms – and asked to describe trends, draw conclusions and suggest improvements. This type of station assesses your ability to handle data logically and communicate findings clearly.

Panel interviews

Although MMIs are now the dominant format, a few veterinary schools still use, or include elements of, panel interviews. In a panel interview, you'll sit with two or three interviewers, usually including academic staff, practising vets or admissions tutors.

Panel interviews allow for longer discussions and can be less stressful if you prefer to build rapport over time. However, because the questions are more predictable, there is a temptation to memorise model answers. Interviewers can usually tell when this happens, so focus on giving thoughtful, genuine responses that draw on your own experiences.

Preparing for your veterinary school interview

Experience shows that personal qualities are just as important as academic ability, and perhaps even more so. The way you come across at interview will depend greatly on how confident and well prepared you are. Confidence based on solid preparation is far better than overconfidence. Many applicants assume they can think on their feet and improvise during the interview, but this approach rarely works. Thorough preparation will not only help you answer expected questions clearly but will also give you the poise to handle unexpected ones calmly.

While interviewers will aim to put you at ease, there will naturally be some tension, and that's no bad thing. A little adrenaline can help you perform at your best. Think of the interview as a professional conversation, where preparation allows your true self and enthusiasm for the course to shine through.

1. Start with your application

Begin by re-reading your UCAS form, including your personal statement and any additional forms you submitted about your work experience. Interviewers often use these as a starting point for questions, and you should expect to be asked about anything you mentioned, from placements to hobbies. Be honest and familiar with every example you've given.

It's also useful to look back over your work experience notes or journals, as selectors may ask you to reflect on specific cases or moments that shaped your understanding of the profession. Focus on what you learnt, rather than listing what you did.

2. Research the profession and the course

Being well-informed is one of the best ways to stand out. Keep up to date with:

- current veterinary and animal welfare issues (e.g. antimicrobial resistance, One Health, sustainability, mental health in the profession);
- professional bodies such as the Royal College of Veterinary Surgeons (RCVS) and British Veterinary Association (BVA);
- news articles, Vet Times, RCVS Knowledge and veterinary podcasts.

You should also know why you're applying to each particular university. Explore course structures, styles of teaching, opportunities for clinical exposure and intercalated or research options. Open days, taster events and student blogs are invaluable for understanding a school's ethos and learning environment.

3. Practise communication and reflection

Strong communication skills are vital for any vet. Practise speaking about your experiences out loud, ideally with a teacher, careers adviser or friend, to help you articulate your thoughts clearly and naturally. Focus on structure: describe a situation, what you did, what you learnt and how it developed your interest or skills.

Remember that in MMIs or panel interviews, how you think and communicate often matters as much as the content of your answer. Stay calm, listen carefully to each question and take a moment to think before responding.

4. Review ethical and welfare principles

Expect questions that test your understanding of ethical and welfare issues. Be familiar with:

- the Five Freedoms of animal welfare;
- core ethical principles such as autonomy, beneficence, non-maleficence and justice;
- and current debates, for example, livestock farming, euthanasia or animal testing.

Interviewers are not looking for perfect answers but for evidence of reasoned thinking and compassion.

5. Practise sample questions

Although you can't predict every question, practising a variety of question types helps you prepare well-rounded responses. Think through questions such as:

- Why do you want to study veterinary medicine?
- What did you learn from your work experience?
- What do you think are the biggest challenges facing the veterinary profession today?
- How would you explain a complex diagnosis to a distressed owner?
- What ethical issues might vets face when treating farm animals?

When answering, always relate back to your own experiences, for example, 'During my placement in a small animal practice, I observed...' or 'While working on a dairy farm, I learned...'. This personal reflection makes your answers memorable and authentic.

6. Manage your mindset and practicalities

Interviews can be nerve-wracking, but preparation helps build genuine confidence.

- **Stay positive**: remember that an invitation to interview means you're a serious contender.
- **Prepare your logistics**: if your interview is in person, plan your route and arrive early. For online interviews, test your camera, microphone and background in advance.
- **Rest and recharge**: good sleep, hydration and a balanced meal beforehand make a noticeable difference to your focus.

7. During the interview

From the moment you enter the room (or join the video call), interviewers are assessing how you communicate and present yourself. Greet them politely, smile and maintain open body language. Listen carefully to questions, and if you don't understand something, ask for clarification rather than guessing.

If you are faced with a question you can't answer, it's perfectly acceptable to say, 'I'm not sure, but I think it might be because...' and explain your reasoning. Interviewers value logical thought processes more than perfect knowledge.

Finally, treat every question as an opportunity to show curiosity, empathy and professionalism – the qualities that make a great future vet.

To help you prepare, Table 3 summarises the main themes that veterinary school interviews tend to explore and suggests how you might structure your answers with confidence.

How to succeed in the interview

Preparing for your interview should be approached with the same focus and commitment as preparing for an exam. Start by revisiting your personal statement and any work experience forms, as these are often the starting point for interview questions. Make sure you can recall specific examples, reflect on what you learnt and explain how these experiences confirmed your motivation to study veterinary medicine.

Next, refresh your knowledge of current issues in veterinary science. Revisit any articles, podcasts or case studies you've explored, and be ready to discuss recent developments such as antimicrobial resistance, sustainability or animal welfare legislation. Above all, be honest – interviewers will quickly notice if something you mention in your statement isn't genuine.

Practice makes perfect

A mock interview is one of the most effective ways to prepare. Many schools or colleges can arrange these, and you might even ask a teacher or careers adviser to role-play common questions. Avoid memorising fixed answers, as rehearsed responses sound unnatural and make it harder to adapt if the question changes slightly. Instead, practise explaining your thoughts clearly and confidently in your own words.

If possible, record a mock interview to observe your body language, tone and pace. Focus on maintaining eye contact, smiling and speaking clearly – all simple things that make a strong impression.

Table 3 Common themes for veterinary school interview questions and effective answer strategies

Theme	Example question	How to approach it
Motivation and insight	Why do you want to study veterinary medicine?	Avoid clichés like 'I love animals and science'. Instead, link your answer to a specific experience or moment that deepened your interest – for example, observing a case on placement or seeing teamwork between vets and nurses. Highlight how your understanding of the profession has evolved.
	When did you decide you wanted to be a vet?	Use a short, clear story that shows how your motivation developed over time, e.g. early curiosity → school studies → work experience confirming your decision.
	What do you think are the challenges of a veterinary career?	Show realism and maturity. Mention long hours, emotional challenges, financial pressures and ethical dilemmas, but balance these with reasons why the profession remains rewarding.
Work experience and reflection	Tell us about something interesting you saw on placement.	Describe a case or scenario, your role in it, what you observed and what you learnt about animal care, teamwork or communication. Reflect, don't just list tasks.
	What did you learn from shadowing a vet?	Focus on transferable skills, such as communication, empathy, critical thinking and what you learnt about the realities of the profession.
	What did you find most challenging about your work experience?	Choose something constructive (e.g. witnessing euthanasia) and explain how you coped, what it taught you and how it confirmed your commitment.
Ethics and animal welfare	How would you handle a client who couldn't afford treatment for their animal?	Acknowledge both compassion for the owner and your duty of care to the animal. Discuss communication, offering options and seeking advice from senior colleagues.
	What are your views on euthanasia?	Balance empathy and professionalism. Explain that euthanasia can be the kindest option when quality of life is poor. Mention sensitivity to owners and animal welfare principles.
	How do you feel about animals being used in research or for meat production?	Take a reasoned approach, e.g. support when it meets ethical and welfare standards, but recognise moral complexity. Refer to the Five Freedoms or legislation if relevant.

(Continued)

Table 3 (Continued)

Theme	Example question	How to approach it
Communication and teamwork	How would you explain a complex diagnosis to a distressed owner?	Show empathy and clarity. Mention using simple language, checking understanding and allowing time for questions.
	Describe a time when you worked as part of a team.	Use the STAR method (Situation, Task, Action, Result) to show collaboration, listening and leadership.
	How do you cope with conflict or stress?	Reflect honestly on a time you managed pressure, for example, balancing studies and work experience, and how you developed resilience.
Academic and scientific knowledge	Why do vets need to study chemistry and physics?	Explain their role in pharmacology, imaging and physiology. Link to examples from your A level studies.
	Tell us about something you've read or researched related to veterinary medicine.	Reference a recent article, journal piece or scientific development and explain why it interested you. Demonstrate curiosity and independent learning.
Current issues and professional awareness	What are the biggest challenges facing the veterinary profession?	Mention workforce shortages, rising client expectations, animal welfare, sustainability and mental health. Support your answer with evidence or examples.
	What does the 'One Health' concept mean?	Explain that human, animal and environmental health are interconnected. Give examples such as antimicrobial resistance or zoonotic diseases.
	What are your thoughts on badger culling and bovine TB?	Show you understand the issue from multiple perspectives – farmers, vets, government policy and animal welfare. Emphasise evidence-based reasoning and compassion.

At the end of your interview

In panel interviews, you may be invited to ask a question at the end (this is not typically part of an MMI). If you do ask something, make sure it is genuine and thoughtful, rather than designed to impress. Avoid questions whose answers are already available on the university website, such as:

- What is the structure of the first year of the course?
- When will I first have contact with animals?

These questions suggest you haven't researched the course thoroughly. If you genuinely have no further questions, it's perfectly acceptable, and professional, to close the interview politely by saying:

'Thank you very much for your time. I've been able to find answers to my questions on the university website and from the students I've spoken to, so there's nothing further from me – it's been great to learn more about the course.'

Smile, thank the panel and leave the interview confidently and courteously.

General interview tips

First impressions count. How you present yourself, through your appearance, speech and body language, can have just as much impact as what you say. Admissions tutors are looking for applicants who can one day represent the veterinary profession, so aim to project confidence, professionalism and warmth.

Body language

- **Smile and make eye contact** when greeting the interviewer, but avoid staring.
- **Sit upright** with open, relaxed posture – this conveys confidence and engagement.
- **Keep gestures natural:** avoid fidgeting, tapping or crossing your arms tightly.
- **Listen actively:** nod occasionally and show genuine interest in what's being said.
- **Stay calm and composed**: if you lose your train of thought, pause briefly and continue; interviewers appreciate poise under pressure.

Speech and communication

- **Speak clearly and at a measured pace**: nervousness can make people rush – consciously slow down if needed.
- **Avoid filler words** such as 'um', 'like', or 'you know'. Recording mock interviews can help you spot and correct these habits.
- **Use professional language**: avoid slang or overly casual phrasing.
- **Greet and thank the interviewers** politely at the start and end of your interview.
- **Adapt for online interviews**: look at the camera when speaking (to simulate eye contact) and keep your notes out of direct view so that you appear attentive.

Dress and appearance

- **Dress smartly and simply**: business or smart-casual attire is appropriate; for example, a shirt or blouse with dark trousers or a skirt or a smart dress.
- **Be comfortable but professional**: you don't need a suit, but avoid anything too casual (e.g. jeans, trainers or hoodies).
- **Online interviews**: check that your background is tidy and well lit. Test your microphone and camera beforehand.

How you are selected

During your interview, whether a Multiple Mini Interview (MMI) or a panel interview, each interviewer will assess you against a set of defined criteria. These typically include communication skills, motivation for the course, problem-solving ability, ethical awareness and suitability for the veterinary profession.

Each interviewer follows structured marking guidelines to ensure that all candidates are assessed fairly and consistently. The scoring systems differ slightly between universities, but most veterinary schools will set a minimum threshold that applicants must meet across all stations or sections to be considered for an offer.

If your score is just below the cut-off, you may be placed on an official or informal waiting list. Final offers are then made once all interviews have been completed and the overall cohort has been ranked.

If you are successful, you will receive a conditional offer, which will also appear on your UCAS Hub account. This usually depends on achieving specific A level grades (most commonly AAA) and meeting any additional non-academic conditions such as health checks, vaccination records or Disclosure and Barring Service (DBS) clearance. Applicants who already hold the required qualifications may receive an unconditional offer.

If you are not successful, you will receive a notification from UCAS once the university has made its decision. While disappointing, this does not mean the end of the road – many strong candidates reapply successfully the following year. You can contact the admissions team to request feedback; some universities will offer personalised comments, while others may only provide general advice. Use any feedback constructively to strengthen your application for future cycles.

What happens next?

Once all of your universities have made their decisions, UCAS will notify you via UCAS Hub. You'll then have a limited period to respond and decide which offer(s) to accept.

If you have one offer

You can either:

- **accept the offer** and focus on meeting the conditions (usually your A level grades); or
- **decline the offer** if you've changed your mind about that university.

If you decide not to accept, you can apply again the following year or use UCAS Extra to apply for alternative courses. However, it is rare for veterinary medicine places to appear through UCAS Extra, so reapplying the next cycle is often the more realistic route.

If you have more than one offer

You must choose:

- a **firm choice** – the university you most want to attend;
- an **insurance choice** – a back-up option, usually with slightly lower entry requirements.

Be careful not to pick your lower offer as your firm choice simply because it seems safer. You are obliged to attend your firm choice if you meet the conditions, and cannot switch to your insurance choice if your firm offer accepts you. You can only take up your insurance offer if your firm choice does not confirm your place.

Even if you narrowly miss the grades required by your firm offer, it's worth remembering that universities occasionally still accept applicants who fall just short of their conditions, particularly if they performed well at interview.

If you receive no offers

If you don't receive any offers, don't panic – many applicants succeed on a second attempt. You have a few options:

- **Reapply the following year** with your achieved grades and additional experience.
- **Pursue a related degree first**, such as bioveterinary science, and consider graduate-entry veterinary medicine later.

Whatever your outcome, use any feedback provided by the veterinary schools to strengthen your application for the next time.

> **Case study**
>
> Amira is about to start her fourth year of the BVMSci Veterinary Medicine and Science course at the University of Surrey. She recently completed her first rotations at the university's network of partner practices.
>
> 'I grew up on the outskirts of Manchester, miles away from any farms, so I always worried that I'd be at a disadvantage applying to vet school. I've wanted to be a vet for as long as I can remember, but it wasn't until sixth form that I realised just how competitive it would be. I knew I needed to show genuine motivation and a realistic understanding of the profession.
>
> 'I started by arranging a few short placements through my local small animal clinic, and from there I gradually built connections. I helped with lambing on a local college farm, volunteered at an RSPCA shelter, and completed the online Vet Widening Participation Virtual Work Experience programme. Keeping a journal of what I'd seen and learned helped me massively when it came to writing my UCAS answers.
>
> 'I chose Surrey because of its modern facilities and the mix of campus life and clinical experience. The first couple of years were intense, but I've learned so much, from anatomy labs to case discussions with real clients during rotations. What surprised me most was how much communication and empathy matter. Vets don't just treat animals; they support owners too.
>
> 'If I could give one piece of advice to applicants, it would be: start early and make every experience count. Whether it's virtual learning, animal volunteering or part-time work, you'll always have something valuable to reflect on. And don't panic if you're not from a farming background – passion, perseverance and genuine curiosity will take you a long way.'

Topical and controversial issues

At interview, the panel won't just want to hear that you love animals – they'll want to know that you understand the real issues vets face in their day-to-day work. This might mean talking about animal welfare, disease outbreaks, sustainability or how wider events such as Brexit or climate change affect the profession. These questions are your chance to show that you think carefully about current events and understand how science, ethics and society overlap in veterinary work.

You don't need to be an expert. What matters is that you can explain an issue clearly, see more than one side of the argument and back up your ideas with a few facts or examples. Interviewers want to see curiosity, common sense and balance, not perfect answers.

How to approach a topical question

If you're asked about a current issue:

1. **Briefly explain what it is** – what's happening and who it affects.
2. **Outline the key points** – why it matters for animals, owners, vets or the wider public.
3. **Show both sides** – what are the benefits, challenges or ethical dilemmas?
4. **Finish with your view** – summarise what you think and why, showing that you've thought it through.

Practising short, structured answers like this will help you stay calm and confident in the interview.

Staying up to date

You can keep track of veterinary news by following:

- **The British Veterinary Association (BVA)** – www.bva.co.uk
- **The Royal College of Veterinary Surgeons (RCVS)** – www.rcvs.org.uk
- **Defra (Department for Environment, Food and Rural Affairs)** – www.gov.uk/defra
- Reputable news outlets or the science/health pages of newspapers.

Try to read a few short articles each week and keep notes on topics that interest you – it makes revision easier later.

Examples of current topics

The issues below are just some of the subjects you might be asked about. You don't need to know them all, but you should be aware of a few and be able to talk about them sensibly.

Animal health and disease

- avian influenza (bird flu) and its effect on wild and farmed birds;
- bluetongue and Epizootic Haemorrhagic Disease (EHD) in livestock;
- African Swine Fever (ASF) in Europe and UK biosecurity measures;
- bovine Tuberculosis (bTB) and badgers.

Farming, food and the environment

- sustainable and intensive farming;
- antibiotic resistance (AMR) and responsible medicine use;
- climate change and its impact on animal health;
- farmgate milk prices and food-chain pressures.

Companion animals and welfare

- breeding and health concerns in flat-faced breeds;
- the XL Bully ban and the Dangerous Dogs Act;
- raw feeding and pet health risks;
- obesity in pets and promoting healthy lifestyles.

The veterinary profession

- the use of animals in research and testing;
- vets' mental health and workload;
- telemedicine and online consultations;
- the impact of Brexit on veterinary work and animal travel.

> **TIP!**
>
> There's rarely a single 'correct' answer to these questions. Interviewers are far more interested in how you think and communicate than in whether you know every detail. Keep your answers balanced, logical and enthusiastic – it shows you've done your research and that you genuinely care about the profession you're hoping to join.

Avian influenza (bird flu)

Avian influenza, often called bird flu, is a viral disease that affects many species of birds, including both poultry and wild birds. It's caused by influenza A viruses such as H5N1, which can spread quickly between flocks and sometimes infect other animals, including people who have close contact with birds.

Since 2020, the UK and Europe have faced their worst outbreaks on record, with large numbers of wild and captive birds affected. Whole colonies of seabirds, such as gannets and skuas, have been hit hard, raising concerns about long-term population losses. For poultry keepers, outbreaks can be devastating – birds must be humanely culled to stop the spread, and strict movement controls and housing orders are often introduced to protect other flocks.

Although the virus rarely passes to humans, isolated cases have been reported in people overseas, usually linked to close contact with infected birds. A few mammals, such as otters and foxes, have also tested positive after eating infected carcasses. More recently, a related H5N1 strain was found in dairy cattle in the United States, reminding vets how adaptable these viruses can be.

For UK vets, bird flu is an important reminder of the One Health approach – a single disease can affect wildlife, farming and human health all at once. Surveillance, good hygiene and strict biosecurity remain the main defences, while researchers continue to study whether vaccination could help reduce future outbreaks.

Bovine tuberculosis (bTB) and badgers

Bovine tuberculosis, or bTB, is a bacterial disease that mainly affects cattle but can also infect other mammals such as badgers and deer. It spreads through close contact and contaminated environments, and infected animals often have to be slaughtered to stop the disease spreading.

For farmers, bTB causes major financial and emotional strain, while for vets it's a long-term challenge that combines animal health, wildlife management and public policy. For many years, controlling bTB has involved a mix of cattle testing, movement restrictions and, in some areas, badger culling. Culling remains controversial – supporters argue it helps limit disease transmission, while opponents say it is inhumane and that the evidence of effectiveness is mixed.

In recent years, the focus has shifted towards vaccination and better biosecurity. Trials of a new CattleBCG vaccine and a matching DIVA test, which can distinguish between infected and vaccinated animals, are underway across several English farms. If successful, these could allow vaccination of cattle from 2026 onwards, potentially reducing the need for culling.

Bovine TB is a good example of how science, policy and animal welfare often overlap in veterinary work. When discussing this topic, try to show that you understand both sides of the argument – the importance of protecting livelihoods and animal welfare, and the need for evidence-based, sustainable solutions.

Vector-borne and emerging livestock diseases

Diseases such as bluetongue and Epizootic Haemorrhagic Disease (EHD) are caused by viruses spread by biting midges, rather than direct animal contact. They mainly affect cattle, sheep and other ruminants, and are becoming more common in northern Europe as climate change allows the midges that carry them to survive in new areas.

Bluetongue, which can cause fever, mouth ulcers and lameness in sheep, has reappeared in the UK several times since it was first detected here in 2007. The most recent cases, caused by the BTV-3 strain, were found in Kent in late 2023 and again in 2024. The infection poses no risk to humans but can lead to significant losses for farmers through animal illness, trade restrictions and culling.

A closely related virus, Epizootic Haemorrhagic Disease (EHD), first appeared in Europe in 2022 and affects cattle and deer in a similar way.

The UK remains officially free of EHD, but its arrival in nearby countries highlights the importance of biosecurity, surveillance and vaccination research.

For aspiring vets, these diseases show how changing weather patterns, global trade and animal movement are reshaping disease risks – a clear example of the One Health and climate resilience principles at work in modern veterinary medicine.

Canine influenza

Canine influenza is a contagious respiratory infection in dogs, caused by influenza A viruses similar to those that affect humans and other animals. The main strains are H3N8, which originally came from horses, and H3N2, which came from birds. Both cause coughing, sneezing, fever and nasal discharge, symptoms that can look very similar to kennel cough.

The disease has become established in the United States and parts of Asia, where outbreaks occasionally occur in kennels and shelters. Most dogs recover fully, but a small number may develop pneumonia, particularly older dogs or those with other health problems. Vaccines are available in countries where the virus is common, although they are not routinely used in the UK, where no cases have been confirmed.

While canine influenza does not infect humans, it's a good reminder of how viruses can jump between species and adapt to new hosts, a concept central to One Health and disease-surveillance work in the veterinary profession.

MRSA

Antimicrobial resistance (AMR) happens when bacteria or other microbes evolve so that antibiotics no longer work effectively against them. It's one of the biggest challenges facing both human and veterinary medicine, and it highlights how closely linked the health of people and animals can be.

In farming, antibiotics are sometimes used to prevent or treat disease in herds and flocks, but overuse can encourage resistant bacteria to develop. The UK has made strong progress in tackling this: sales of antibiotics for food-producing animals have fallen by almost 60% since 2014. Vets now focus on prevention through vaccination, biosecurity and herd management rather than routine treatment.

A well-known example of AMR is MRSA (*Methicillin-Resistant Staphylococcus aureus*), a 'superbug' first recognised in hospitals but also occasionally found in pets and horses. In most cases, animals pick up MRSA from humans, and the infection risk to people is very low. Even so, it reminds vets how important hygiene, infection control and careful prescribing are in all clinical settings.

For interview purposes, AMR is a key topic because it combines science, ethics and public health, showing how vets protect both animal welfare and human safety by using medicines responsibly.

Foot-and-mouth disease

Foot-and-mouth disease (FMD) is a highly contagious viral illness that affects cattle, pigs, sheep and other cloven-hoofed animals. It spreads through saliva, milk and dung, and can even travel long distances on the wind or on contaminated vehicles and clothing. Although it doesn't infect people, an outbreak can have devastating effects on farming and animal welfare.

The UK's most serious outbreak occurred in 2001, when millions of animals had to be culled to stop the disease spreading. A smaller incident in 2007, linked to a laboratory leak, was quickly contained. Since then, the UK has remained officially free of FMD, but the virus continues to circulate in parts of Asia, Africa and South America, meaning there is always a small risk of it returning through trade or travel.

If a vet suspects FMD, it must be reported immediately to Defra or the Animal and Plant Health Agency (APHA) as a notifiable disease. Control measures include strict movement restrictions, tracing and sometimes emergency vaccination. Treatment of infected animals is not allowed because of the risk of spreading the virus further.

For students, FMD illustrates how biosecurity, rapid response and clear communication are crucial in protecting animal health and the farming economy, and how vets play a vital role in national disease surveillance.

Bovine spongiform encephalopathy (BSE)

Bovine spongiform encephalopathy, or BSE, is a brain disease in cattle caused by abnormal proteins called prions. It was first recognised in the UK in the 1980s after cattle became infected through feed that contained remains of other animals. The disease damages the brain and nervous system, leading to uncoordinated movement and behavioural changes.

BSE became a major crisis in the 1990s when scientists discovered that a related condition in humans, variant Creutzfeldt–Jakob disease (vCJD), was linked to eating beef from infected animals. Millions of cattle were culled, beef exports were banned for a decade and the outbreak led to major changes in farming and food-safety regulations.

Today, BSE is rare and well controlled. The UK still tests cattle routinely, and feeding animal protein to livestock remains banned. The few cases reported in recent years, such as one in Cornwall in 2023, have been atypical forms that occur naturally in older cattle and are not contagious or dangerous to humans.

The BSE outbreak reshaped the relationship between science, government and the public, showing how vital transparency, traceability and veterinary oversight are for maintaining food safety and trust in the agricultural industry.

Animal obesity

Obesity is now officially recognised as a disease in companion animals and is one of the most common preventable health issues seen in veterinary practice. Recent surveys, such as the PDSA Animal Wellbeing (PAW) Report 2024, suggest that around half of UK dogs and over 40% of cats are overweight or obese.

The causes are often similar to those in humans – too many calories, not enough exercise and a lack of awareness about portion control. Many owners also express affection through food, which can make managing weight difficult. Certain breeds, such as Labradors and pugs, are particularly prone to weight gain.

Excess weight increases the risk of serious health problems, including arthritis, diabetes, heart disease and breathing difficulties, and it can significantly shorten a pet's lifespan.

Vets play an important role in tackling the issue through client education, weight management plans and preventative care, often supported by vet nurses running regular weight-check clinics. For interview purposes, pet obesity is a useful example of how vets combine medical knowledge with communication and behavioural skills to promote long-term animal welfare.

Canine lungworm

Canine lungworm (*Angiostrongylus vasorum*) is a parasitic worm that affects dogs and foxes, living in the heart and blood vessels of the lungs. It's now widespread across the UK and can be life-threatening if left untreated.

The parasite is carried by slugs and snails, and dogs can become infected if they eat them, or even if they come into contact with their slime trails on toys, water bowls or grass. Foxes play a major role in spreading the parasite between regions.

Typical symptoms include coughing, tiredness, unexplained bleeding or bruising and changes in behaviour. In severe cases, lungworm can cause heart and breathing problems. The condition does not affect humans, but it is an important animal welfare and preventative care issue.

Vets diagnose lungworm through faecal or blood tests and treat it using antiparasitic medicines. Preventative treatments are also available and are increasingly recommended year-round, especially as climate change creates milder, wetter conditions that help slugs and snails thrive.

For interview purposes, lungworm is a good example of how disease control, owner education and environmental awareness come together in modern veterinary practice.

Emerging and notifiable diseases

Alongside familiar conditions like lungworm or bovine TB, vets also monitor a range of notifiable and emerging diseases – illnesses that must, by law, be reported to Defra or the Animal and Plant Health Agency (APHA) if suspected. These include rare but serious infections such as swine influenza, anthrax and avian influenza, which can affect both livestock and wildlife.

Although these diseases are uncommon in the UK, they are important examples of how quickly animal health issues can become national or even global concerns. For instance:

- Swine influenza is a viral disease found in pigs that occasionally passes to humans. While usually mild, it shows how viruses can cross species barriers – a reminder of the One Health link between human and animal health.
- Anthrax, caused by the bacterium *Bacillus anthracis*, can survive in soil for decades. It occasionally re-emerges in grazing animals, but strict biosecurity, vaccination and surveillance mean UK cases are now extremely rare.
- Other diseases, such as African Swine Fever, bluetongue and rabies in bats, remain under close monitoring to prevent re-introduction into the UK.

These examples highlight the importance of disease surveillance, rapid reporting and clear communication between vets, farmers, government and the public. They also remind us that veterinary work extends far beyond the consulting room – vets are part of the front line in protecting animal welfare, food security and public health.

Intensive and sustainable farming

The UK produces huge quantities of meat, milk and eggs to meet demand for affordable food, and many farms now rely on intensive production systems to do so. These systems can be highly efficient, but they raise important questions about animal welfare, sustainability and ethics.

Veterinary professionals play a crucial role in helping farmers balance productivity with welfare standards, advising on housing, nutrition, biosecurity and disease prevention. The rise of large-scale pig and poultry units (sometimes called 'mega farms') has also made public concern about welfare and environmental impact more prominent, particularly around issues such as live exports, confinement and humane slaughter.

Following Brexit, the UK's Agriculture Act 2020 introduced new support schemes that reward farmers for producing food sustainably and improving animal welfare, rather than simply for the amount they produce. Vets are key partners in this transition, helping to ensure that farming remains both economically viable and ethically responsible.

Antibiotic resistance

A major challenge linked to intensive farming is the use of antibiotics in livestock. These medicines are vital for treating illness, but overuse can lead to antimicrobial resistance (AMR), when bacteria evolve to survive antibiotic treatment. Resistant strains, such as certain types of *E. coli* or *Salmonella*, can spread between animals, people and the environment, making infections harder to treat.

The UK has made major progress: sales of antibiotics for food-producing animals have fallen by nearly 60% since 2014, and growth-promoting antibiotics are no longer used. Current efforts focus on disease prevention rather than routine medication, using tools such as vaccination, better housing and improved hygiene.

AMR is a clear example of the One Health approach, where human, animal and environmental health are linked. Vets play a central role in safeguarding antibiotics through responsible prescribing and farmer education, ensuring these life-saving drugs remain effective for both animals and people.

Animal ethics and fox hunting

Vets are often at the centre of public debates about how animals are used or managed, from farm production to field sports. One long-standing example is fox hunting, which was banned in England and Wales by the Hunting Act 2004 and in Scotland by newer legislation in 2023.

Supporters of hunting view it as part of rural heritage and a method of population control, while opponents see it as cruel and unnecessary. Even though hunting with dogs is now illegal, limited exemptions allow up to two dogs to flush a wild mammal to be shot for pest control or conservation purposes.

For applicants, this topic is less about taking a particular stance and more about showing you can see both sides of an ethical question. Vets must constantly weigh up welfare, practicality and public expectation, for example, when advising on wildlife management, euthanasia or animal use in sport.

A good interview answer might discuss how laws such as the Animal Welfare Act 2006 aim to protect animals from suffering, while also recognising that different people define welfare and necessity in different ways. What matters most is being able to discuss the issue reasonably, knowledgeably and respectfully.

Dog breeds, welfare and the law

Some of the most debated animal welfare topics in the UK involve dog ownership and breeding. Two major areas to be aware of are the Dangerous Dogs Act and the High Profile Breeds (HPB) list.

The Dangerous Dogs Act (1991) was introduced to reduce attacks by certain types of dogs. It bans the breeding, sale or exchange of specified breeds, including the Pit Bull Terrier, Japanese Tosa, Dogo Argentino, Fila Brasileiro, and, since 2024, the American XL Bully.

Existing XL Bullies may still be kept, but owners must follow strict conditions – they must be registered, neutered, microchipped, muzzled in public and kept on a lead. Breaching these conditions can result in prosecution and seizure of the dog.

While designed to protect the public, breed-specific legislation remains controversial. Many animal welfare organisations, including the British Veterinary Association (BVA) and the RSPCA, argue that a dog's behaviour depends more on training, socialisation and owner responsibility than breed alone. For vets, this raises ethical and professional questions – for instance, what to do if asked to euthanise a banned breed that has shown no aggression.

Separately, the Kennel Club's High Profile Breeds list highlights breeds with known health or welfare problems, such as pugs, bulldogs and German shepherds. These dogs are often prone to conditions like breathing difficulties or spinal deformities due to selective breeding for exaggerated features. The aim is not to discourage ownership, but to encourage responsible breeding and better health screening.

Together, these examples show the complex balance between public safety, animal welfare and owner education. In interviews, you could use them to demonstrate that being a vet isn't just about medicine – it's also about understanding ethics, law and the relationship between people and their animals.

Breeding, science and ethics

Hybrid and designer dogs

Over the past two decades, there has been a boom in so-called designer crossbreeds – combinations such as Labradoodles, Cockapoos and

Cavapoos. These dogs are often bred for appearance, temperament or claims of being 'hypoallergenic'. While some crosses can combine positive traits from both parents, others suffer from inherited health or behavioural problems if breeding is poorly managed.

Most welfare organisations, including the British Veterinary Association (BVA) and the Kennel Club, stress that good breeding practice and health testing matter far more than whether a dog is pedigree or crossbreed. Problems arise when popular crosses are bred quickly to meet demand, sometimes by unlicensed breeders or puppy farms, without appropriate health screening.

This topic often appears in interviews because it raises ethical questions about how humans prioritise looks, trends and profit over welfare. A thoughtful answer might consider the role of vets in educating owners, supporting responsible breeders and promoting adoption from shelters rather than impulse buying.

Animal testing and research

The use of animals in scientific research remains a sensitive and often misunderstood topic. In the UK, such work is strictly regulated under the Animals (Scientific Procedures) Act 1986, which requires any use of animals for research or teaching to be justified, licensed and reviewed for welfare standards.

Researchers must follow the '3Rs' principle:

- **Replacement** (using alternatives such as cell cultures or computer models wherever possible).
- **Reduction** (using the smallest number of animals necessary).
- **Refinement** (minimising pain and distress).

Animals are mainly used in medical, veterinary and pharmaceutical research that cannot yet be replicated by other methods. This work has contributed to vaccines, anaesthetics and new treatments that benefit both humans and animals.

For aspiring vets, this issue demonstrates the ethical balance between animal welfare and scientific progress. It's not about defending or condemning research, but showing you understand why it's tightly controlled, why alternatives are encouraged and how vets help to ensure humane, ethical standards are met in every setting.

Dairy farming and market pressures

The UK is one of the largest milk producers in Europe, supplying around 90% of its own demand. Yet dairy farmers face ongoing challenges from fluctuating prices, rising costs and changing consumer expectations.

After Brexit, the cost of exporting dairy products and sourcing labour increased, while the war in Ukraine and global inflation pushed up feed and energy prices. At the same time, supermarkets compete to keep retail prices low, meaning that many farmers' profit margins remain extremely tight. Some have left the industry, while others have adapted by producing higher-welfare or more sustainable milk, or by creating value-added products such as cheese or yoghurt.

For vets, the health of the dairy sector matters not just economically but ethically. When prices are low, there can be pressure to cut corners on housing, nutrition or preventative care, so vets play a vital role in helping farmers maintain welfare and sustainability even when financial conditions are tough.

This topic also links closely with issues such as food security, sustainability and animal welfare standards, which are all good areas to discuss in interviews.

Brexit and the veterinary profession

Since the UK left the European Union, vets have found themselves at the centre of many of the changes affecting animals, farming and food production. Brexit has influenced everything from animal movement and export certification to labour availability, welfare standards and research funding.

One of the biggest changes has been the increased need for Official Veterinarians (OVs) to certify exports of meat, dairy and live animals to the EU. This has created new opportunities for vets in public health and regulatory roles, but has also placed pressure on workforce capacity.

Labour shortages in abattoirs and farms, as well as higher costs for transport and compliance, have affected food production and trade. Meanwhile, animal welfare and environmental rules have remained broadly in line with EU standards, though the UK now sets its own targets through policies like the Agriculture Act 2020 and Animal Health and Welfare Pathway.

Brexit has also had an impact on research and veterinary education, with the UK rejoining the Horizon Europe programme in 2023 to support international collaboration.

For aspiring vets, Brexit is a reminder that animal health doesn't exist in isolation – it's shaped by politics, trade and international cooperation. Understanding how policy decisions influence welfare, farming and the veterinary workforce shows awareness of the wider context in which vets work.

COVID-19 and One Health

The COVID-19 pandemic was a powerful reminder of how closely human, animal and environmental health are connected. Caused by the coronavirus SARS-CoV-2, it is thought to have originated from an animal source before spreading between people across the world.

Although the virus mainly affects humans, some animals, including cats, dogs and farmed mink, have tested positive, usually after contact with infected people. These cases were rare, but they highlighted the need for good hygiene, surveillance and communication between medical and veterinary professionals.

During the pandemic, many vets played an active role in maintaining animal welfare and food safety under difficult conditions. Some worked in diagnostic labs processing human COVID-19 tests; others helped manage the welfare of animals when owners were isolating.

For future vets, COVID-19 illustrates why the One Health approach matters so much. It shows how disease can cross species, how global cooperation is essential and how veterinary expertise contributes not only to animal care but also to public health and pandemic preparedness.

The importance of One Health

You might notice that many of the issues vets deal with, from bird flu to antibiotic resistance, link animals, people and the environment. This idea is known as One Health. It recognises that the health of humans, animals and ecosystems are all connected, and that problems in one area can quickly affect the others.

A good example is Ebola virus disease, which is thought to have spread to people through contact with infected wildlife such as fruit bats and primates in parts of Africa. While it doesn't affect UK animals, it shows how diseases that begin in animals can have a major impact on human health. The same is true of more familiar examples such as COVID-19 and avian influenza.

Vets play a key role in this global picture – not just treating sick animals, but helping to monitor diseases, protect public health and promote sustainable farming and wildlife conservation. Having a broad awareness of One Health will help you understand how the profession fits into the wider world and why global events often feature in veterinary news.

Other issues

In addition to the topics already covered, it's helpful for aspiring vets to have a broad awareness of other animal diseases that are monitored in the UK and around the world. Some of these are *notifiable*, meaning any suspected case must be reported to Defra or the Animal and Plant Health Agency (APHA). Others are *emerging diseases* that could spread to the UK through trade, climate change or wildlife movement.

Recent examples highlighted by Defra and the World Organisation for Animal Health (WOAH) include:

- **African horse sickness** – a serious midge-borne disease of horses; never recorded in the UK but present in parts of Europe.
- **African Swine Fever** – affects pigs and wild boar; widespread in parts of continental Europe but not present in the UK.
- **West Nile virus** – carried by mosquitoes and wild birds; occasionally seen in southern Europe, posing risks to both horses and humans.
- **Koi herpesvirus disease** – affects carp and koi; outbreaks have occurred in UK fisheries.
- **Rabies in bats** – very rare but still detected occasionally in the UK.

You do not need to memorise every disease or date. Instead, focus on understanding how vets help detect, report and control outbreaks, and why surveillance matters for protecting animal welfare, trade and public health.

To keep up to date, visit:

- Defra: notifiable diseases in animals: www.gov.uk/guidance/notifiable-diseases-in-animals
- World Organisation for Animal Health (WOAH): www.woah.org/en/what-we-do/animal-health-and-welfare/animal-diseases

Checking these sites before your interview will show that you're well-informed and proactive, qualities that admissions tutors look for in future vets.

Climate change and sustainable veterinary practice

Climate change is one of the biggest challenges facing animal health today. Rising temperatures, extreme weather events and changing ecosystems are already affecting livestock, wildlife and companion animals. Heat stress, new vector-borne diseases and disruptions to food supply all have direct impacts on animal welfare.

Vets are increasingly involved in developing sustainable approaches to farming, transport and practice management, from reducing emissions and antibiotic use to improving waste management and energy efficiency in clinics. Organisations such as the BVA and Vet Sustain encourage vets to adopt 'greener practice' principles, and the RCVS Knowledge initiative now includes sustainability in its quality-improvement framework.

For interviews, it's useful to think about the vet's dual role: protecting animal health while also supporting sustainable, environmentally responsible practice.

Selective breeding and animal welfare

Selective breeding remains one of the most debated welfare topics in the UK. Flat-faced (brachycephalic) breeds such as French bulldogs and pugs often suffer from chronic respiratory and eye problems caused by their exaggerated features. The BVA, RCVS and animal welfare charities have called for greater public awareness and changes in breeding standards.

Advances in genetics also raise new ethical questions. Gene editing in livestock could improve disease resistance or productivity, but it must be balanced against welfare and consumer confidence. When discussing this topic, focus on how vets can advise owners and breeders responsibly, promote animal welfare and support evidence-based policies rather than extreme views on either side.

Workforce wellbeing and mental health

The wellbeing of veterinary professionals has become a major concern in recent years. High workloads, client expectations, financial pressures and emotional demands can all take a toll. Surveys by the BVA, Vetlife and the Mind Matters Initiative (RCVS) show that vets experience higher levels of stress and burnout than many other professions.

In response, vet schools and employers are placing greater emphasis on mental health support, teamwork and work–life balance. Universities now teach resilience, communication skills and self-care as part of professional-skills training. When preparing for interview, it's useful to understand that modern veterinary practice values compassion and wellbeing just as much as scientific ability.

Food security and the global role of vets

Feeding a growing global population while maintaining high welfare and environmental standards is one of the biggest challenges of the 21st century. Vets play a key role in ensuring safe, sustainable and ethical food production, from preventing disease outbreaks in livestock to monitoring animal welfare and supporting biosecurity in international trade.

Events such as the COVID-19 pandemic, the spread of avian influenza and the ongoing threat of African Swine Fever have shown how animal health, human health and food systems are deeply interconnected. This is the essence of the One Health approach: recognising that healthy animals contribute directly to healthy people and a healthy planet.

In interviews, it's useful to show awareness that the role of a vet extends far beyond clinical practice. Veterinary professionals contribute to public health, food safety, research and global disease control, helping to secure the future of sustainable agriculture and responsible food systems worldwide.

Topical issues summary

Veterinary medicine doesn't exist in isolation – it's part of a wider network that connects animal health, human wellbeing, the environment and society. From global diseases such as avian influenza and bovine tuberculosis to issues like pet obesity, sustainable farming and antimicrobial resistance, the challenges facing the profession are constantly changing.

Admissions tutors don't expect you to be an expert, but they do expect you to be curious, informed and thoughtful. Keeping up to date with the latest developments through Defra, the British Veterinary Association (BVA) and reliable news sources will help you understand how science, ethics and policy intersect in real life.

When these topics arise in an interview, focus on showing awareness and reasoning, not on memorising facts. Demonstrate that you can look at both sides of an argument, whether it's about vaccination policy, farming ethics or wildlife management, and explain your view clearly and logically.

Above all, remember that these issues reflect what being a vet is really about: combining scientific knowledge with compassion, integrity and communication skills to protect both animals and the wider world.

> **Case study**
>
> Marie grew up around horses, and had always had her sights set on being an equine vet. She went on to qualify as a veterinary surgeon after studying at the University of Bristol, but after adopting two corn snakes, she got hooked on exotics! Having completed some placements in exotics practices and zoos, she knew this was the path for her, and now works as an exotics and zoo vet.
>
> 'After graduating, I started off working in a small animal and exotics practice that supported me to be competent and confident with consulting, surgery and working with both domestic and exotic animals. The first year was a steep learning curve, but I had some good colleagues to lean on when I needed them. After 18 months, a residency in avian medicine became available in a referral hospital. These specialist training positions are rare, and although I wasn't necessarily excited about birds, I knew this was one of very few chances to get that training. I applied and got the position. I then spent three years specialising, with a high bird caseload that I grew to enjoy, but also a wide range of other exotic animals. I did placements in pathology, ophthalmology, surgery, medicine and did night shifts with small animals as well as the day-to-day work. I completed my certificate in zoo medicine at the same time.

'After my residency, I moved to Birmingham and set up an exotics and zoo department in a practice group, which expanded rapidly and is still thriving. I completed my diploma in zoo and wildlife medicine while there and became an accredited specialist. After six years, I was struggling to run a large, busy department and keep up with being a parent and having a life outside work, so I switched to consultancy work. I spent a couple of years as a visiting specialist to various zoo collections and practices, wrote articles, took on RSPCA cases with exotics animals and started writing a textbook on exotic animal medicine and surgery. I enjoyed the freedom and flexibility to pick and choose what I wanted to do. However, when a full-time zoo job came up locally, I couldn't resist it; I went on to spend three years working with a huge range of species, from invertebrates to rhinos. I also finished my textbook, somehow! I now work part-time for an exotics practice, continuing consultancy work and writing around this.

'My current role is as head vet for an exotics practice, consulting and operating for three days a week and covering emergencies. The days are long and busy, but I enjoy having a hands-on role and being able to build up relationships with clients and pets, and investigate and treat cases to a high standard. We work with zoo collections as well as private keepers, so the patients vary greatly and I love the unpredictability and the range of skills needed to successfully handle and treat them. I have a range of interests, including reptile surgery, invertebrate medicine, reproductive management in zoo mammals and legal work.

'The most rewarding part of the job is that I can actually make a difference to an animal or their carer's day, or even life. It is a very tough job a lot of the time, but at the end of the day when I reflect on what we have achieved, it feels good. I love completing a new or challenging surgery, and seeing an animal that was struggling return to full health.

'There is a huge weight of expectation on vets to be able to fix animals immediately and with cost limitations. With exotic patients, these issues are often compounded by the lack of knowledge available for many species and disease processes, so there is a constant learning process and daily challenges. Financial restrictions are also more common with many exotic and zoo animals, so trying to reach a diagnosis and cure can be a careful balancing act, and as a profession, we are not good at accepting defeat and take personal responsibility for not achieving success regardless of limitations that have been placed on us.

'There is a growing acceptance that the way vet practices work is not good for the mental and physical health of vets – 12-hour days, being called in overnight and on days off, a constant stream of new patients with restricted time to deal with them, higher pet-owner demands (and increased social media expression of discontent) plus greater financial pressures and lack of support have led to the loss of many good vets from the profession. The recognition that this is not a constructive way to work is a big step forward, and working conditions are slowly changing for the better.

> 'If you are an aspiring vet, be prepared to work incredibly hard, not only for exam results and to gain experience now, but throughout the degree and in working life, especially that first year when everything is new and scary. Make sure you have a good support network of friends and family who are happy to provide tea, cake and listen to you vent when you've had a rough day. It is a career that is going to push you to your limits repeatedly, but it's also a profession where you are surrounded by people that understand your battles, will help you wherever they can and be like a family you never expected!
>
> 'Oh, and be prepared to end up with a house full of stray or slightly wonky pets that have nowhere else to go!'

Importance of the interview

Being invited to interview is a real achievement – it means your application has made a strong impression, and you're now being given the chance to show who you are beyond your grades and work experience. The interview is your opportunity to demonstrate your enthusiasm for veterinary medicine, your ability to think critically about issues and your awareness of what the profession involves.

A confident, well-prepared interview can make a real difference. Admissions tutors often reconsider candidates who perform strongly at interview, even if their grades later fall slightly short of their offer conditions. The key is to show that you have the curiosity, judgement and communication skills that make a great vet.

A successful interview isn't about knowing everything; it's about showing how you think, how you communicate and how you learn. Reflect on what you've read in this chapter, keep up with current veterinary issues and approach your interview with genuine interest and self-awareness. Those qualities are exactly what admissions tutors, and future clients, are looking for.

> **Fact**: Dogs can alert their owners of an epileptic seizure up to an hour before it occurs.

8 | A leopard does not change its spots
Non-standard applicants

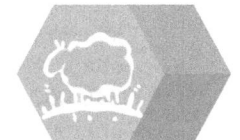

Most of this book has focused on applicants following the typical UK school-leaver route, studying A levels, the International Baccalaureate (IB), Scottish Highers or the Irish Leaving Certificate. However, these are not the only pathways into veterinary medicine.

Every year, vet schools receive applications from a wide range of candidates, including mature students, graduates, international applicants and those with vocational or alternative qualifications. Many universities also offer Foundation or Gateway programmes for students who show strong potential but do not meet the standard academic entry requirements.

If you don't fit the traditional profile, don't be discouraged – there are multiple routes into the profession, and veterinary schools actively encourage diverse backgrounds and experiences. The next sections outline the main alternative-entry options and offer advice on how to strengthen your application, whatever your starting point.

International and EU applicants

Competition for veterinary places is strong, but every UK vet school welcomes international students. If you're applying from outside the UK, it's a good idea to contact admissions tutors early to confirm that your qualifications meet entry requirements and to discuss any additional guidance for overseas applicants.

Even if you haven't taken A levels or the International Baccalaureate (IB), universities accept a wide range of international qualifications, from Advanced Placements (APs) to local high-school diplomas, provided they are recognised as equivalent. You can check this using UCAS, UK ENIC or your local British Council office.

Tuition fees and scholarships

International students (including EU nationals without UK settled status) pay the full overseas tuition fee, typically between £38,000 and £46,000 per year for veterinary courses. Fees vary by university and are reviewed annually.

Many vet schools offer international scholarships or bursaries, and it's worth researching these early through each university's website. You apply for these directly, not through UCAS. Further information on funding can be found in Chapter 10.

English-language requirements

If English is not your first language, you'll need to demonstrate proficiency through an accepted test. Most universities require:

- **IELTS Academic:** minimum overall score of 7.0 (with no band below 6.5); or
- **TOEFL iBT:** around 100 overall (with no section below 23).

Some universities also accept the Pearson PTE Academic or Cambridge English (C1 Advanced). If you haven't completed the test before applying, it can usually form part of a conditional offer.

Visas

All international students (except Irish citizens or EU students with pre-settled or settled status) must hold a Student Visa before starting the course. Once you have an offer, your university will issue a CAS (Confirmation of Acceptance for Studies), which you'll need to apply for the visa. You'll also need to provide financial documentation and proof of English proficiency. Visa processing times vary, so start the process as early as possible.

UCAS application

Students applying from outside the UK use the same UCAS system and deadlines as domestic applicants. The two areas that often cause difficulty are the personal statement and academic reference, especially if your teachers are less familiar with UK applications.

Make sure your personal statement focuses on your motivation, relevant experience and understanding of veterinary work rather than general achievements. It can also help to explain why you wish to study in the UK. Your referee should comment on your academic strengths and suitability for a demanding science-based degree, not just personal qualities.

UCAS provides detailed guidance and short videos on both sections – it's worth sharing these resources with your referee before submission.

Work experience

All UK vet schools expect applicants to gain some relevant animal or veterinary experience, even if you're applying from abroad. If in-person placements are difficult to access, you can supplement these with animal-related voluntary work, online courses or virtual placements. If there are genuine barriers to gaining experience, ask your referee to explain this in the reference and describe what you did instead to learn about the profession.

Interviews

Most international interviews are now held online through video conferencing platforms. Occasionally, universities may invite candidates to attend in person in the UK or during overseas recruitment events. It's best to check each school's policy before applying so you can plan accordingly.

Studying outside the UK

Some students choose to study veterinary medicine abroad, either for lifestyle reasons or because places in the UK are limited. Several international veterinary schools now offer programmes taught in English, and some hold RCVS accreditation, meaning their graduates can automatically register to practise in the UK.

Examples include universities in Australia, New Zealand, South Africa, Canada, the United States and the Caribbean (for example, St George's University in Grenada). Other European schools, such as those in Ireland and parts of central Europe, also teach in English and are seeking or hold RCVS approval.

If you're considering this route, always check the RCVS list of accredited veterinary degrees before applying. Graduates from non-accredited programmes can still work in the UK, but they must first pass the Statutory Membership Examination, which assesses clinical and professional competence and is held annually at a UK vet school.

Since Brexit, EU veterinary qualifications are no longer automatically recognised, and graduates from the EU or elsewhere will need to apply for a Skilled Worker Visa to work in the UK.

Further details on accreditation, examinations and registration can be found on the RCVS website (www.rcvs.org.uk).

Mature students

A mature applicant is anyone aged 21 or over when starting the course. Mature and career-change students bring valuable perspectives to veterinary medicine, from previous careers in animal care, research, teaching or completely different fields.

Although competition for places remains high, most UK vet schools actively welcome mature students who can demonstrate academic readiness, motivation and relevant experience. You'll still need to meet the core science entry requirements, but universities may consider alternative qualifications such as Access to HE Diplomas (Science or Veterinary Science), Open University modules or recently completed A levels.

In your personal statement, focus on what has led you to this career change and what you've learnt from previous experiences. Highlight:

- why you want to study veterinary medicine now;
- how you've explored the profession through work experience or volunteering;
- what transferable skills you bring (for example, communication, problem solving, teamwork or resilience).

Your maturity and broader life experience can be real advantages, especially in areas like client communication, decision-making and emotional awareness.

If you're unsure whether your qualifications meet entry requirements, contact admissions tutors directly for advice before applying. Most are happy to discuss your individual background and suggest suitable entry routes, including Foundation or Gateway programmes if you need to build up your academic profile.

Students with disabilities and additional learning needs

All UK veterinary schools welcome applications from students with disabilities, long-term health conditions or specific learning differences such as dyslexia or ADHD. Under the Equality Act 2010, universities have a duty to ensure that students are not disadvantaged and that reasonable adjustments are made to support access, participation and success.

If you have a disability or health condition, it's a good idea to check the course requirements for each university and to contact their Disability or Wellbeing Service early in the application process. This allows them to advise you about available adjustments, for example, accessible teaching spaces, extra time in exams, assistive technology or adjustments during practical and clinical training.

It's helpful to include relevant details on your UCAS application so the university can plan your support in advance. All information is treated confidentially and used only to arrange appropriate adjustments.

Vet schools are committed to supporting a diverse student community and will work with you to ensure you can meet the RCVS Day One Competences safely and effectively. If you have any concerns about meeting practical or physical aspects of the course, admissions staff can discuss these with you in confidence.

For further guidance, contact the individual university's Disability Support Service or visit their website for information about access arrangements, support plans and available funding such as the Disabled Students' Allowance (DSA).

Gateway and Foundation programmes

If you're passionate about becoming a vet but don't meet the standard academic entry requirements, you might still have a route into veterinary medicine through a Gateway or Foundation programme.

These courses are designed for students who have the ability and motivation to succeed but who may have faced barriers to achieving higher grades or accessing work experience. They often consider factors such as your school background, postcode, time spent in care or family circumstances, alongside your academic record.

Most Gateway or Foundation programmes are six years in total, with the first year focusing on core scientific knowledge, study skills and preparation for clinical training. If you meet the required standard in your first year, you progress automatically onto the main veterinary degree.

These routes are now offered at several UK vet schools, including Bristol, Nottingham, Surrey, Glasgow, Harper & Keele, Edinburgh and the Royal Veterinary College. Each programme has its own eligibility criteria and application process, so it's important to check the individual course pages carefully before applying.

Students on these pathways often receive additional academic and pastoral support, and many describe them as an excellent transition into the demands of veterinary study.

If you're unsure whether you qualify, contact the admissions office – they'll be happy to advise you. You can also find details on the UCAS course search under Veterinary Medicine (Gateway/Foundation) or through the British Veterinary Association (BVA) and Vet Schools Council (VSC) websites.

Graduate entry into veterinary medicine

An increasing number of students are choosing to apply to veterinary school after completing another degree. Most graduate applicants hold qualifications in subjects such as biological sciences, zoology, animal science or biomedical science, but some come from completely different backgrounds and bring valuable transferable skills.

UK veterinary schools welcome graduate applicants who can demonstrate strong academic ability, motivation and a clear understanding of the profession. Entry requirements vary between universities, but you'll usually need:

- a 2:i or above in a relevant biological science degree (some may consider a 2:ii with additional experience);
- evidence of recent study in chemistry or biology if your degree is in another field.

Some universities offer accelerated four-year graduate-entry programmes, while others require graduates to complete the full five- or six-year course.

Funding and finance

Graduate applicants are usually not eligible for full undergraduate funding through Student Finance England if they already hold a degree. However, partial support may be available for tuition or living costs, depending on your circumstances. It's important to research alternative funding options, such as university bursaries, postgraduate loans (for certain accelerated routes) or scholarships for graduate-entry students.

Application advice

Graduate applicants apply via UCAS in the same way as school-leavers. In your personal statement, focus on your motivation for changing direction, what you've learnt from previous study or work and how your experience has strengthened your commitment to becoming a vet.

Highlight your relevant scientific background, practical experience and transferable skills such as communication, problem solving and teamwork. Many graduates find that their maturity and perspective make them particularly strong candidates at interview.

Case study

After completing a degree in Biomedical Science, Sophie realised she wanted to return to her first passion – working with animals. Her journey demonstrates how determination and relevant experience can open up a new route into veterinary medicine.

'I always loved animals, but when I left school, I didn't think I had the grades for veterinary medicine. I chose to study Biomedical Science instead and spent three years learning about physiology, microbiology and immunology. During my degree, I realised how much I missed the animal side of biology, so I began volunteering at a local small animal clinic at weekends.

'After graduating, I worked full-time as a veterinary receptionist for two years, which gave me insight into client communication, the realities of practice life, and the teamwork between vets, nurses and support staff. My employers were really supportive – they helped me find opportunities to shadow consultations and observe minor procedures.

'When I decided to apply for veterinary medicine as a graduate, I contacted admissions tutors at several universities to check whether my qualifications met their requirements. I also completed an online chemistry refresher course to strengthen my application.

'The interview process was nerve-wracking, but my previous degree helped me talk confidently about evidence-based practice and critical thinking. I was offered a place on the four-year accelerated graduate-entry programme at the RVC, and I'm now in my second year.

'If I could give one piece of advice to other graduates or career changers, it would be: don't rule yourself out. It might take longer or require a different path, but the experience and maturity you bring are real strengths. The vet schools value diversity, and your journey can be a huge asset.'

Fact: A cat can be either right-pawed or left-pawed.

9 | A bird in the hand
Results day

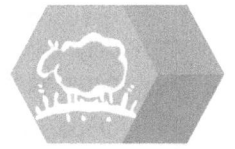

You have done all of the hard work – your personal statement, the interview, the examinations – and you are now waiting for your results, the results that will determine whether you have achieved what you need to take your university place. This chapter explains what happens when you get your results, and, if you have achieved grades that are either better or worse than expected, what other options are available to you.

When the results are available

- A levels – mid-August;
- IB – early in July;
- Scottish Highers – first week of August.

Ask your school or college for the exact date and time that they will issue you with the results. Whichever of the exam systems you are sitting, you need to act quickly if you:

- have missed the grades or scores that you require to satisfy your firm offer;
- are not holding any offers and wish to apply through UCAS Clearing.

What to do if you have no offers: UCAS Extra

If you apply for five courses and either receive no offers or decline all the offers you get, you are eligible for UCAS Extra. Extra operates from the end of February to the beginning of July and allows you to add one additional choice at a time.

To find a course using Extra, use the UCAS search tool and the filter 'Show courses with vacancies'. Next, contact the universities and colleges listed to check if they'll consider you. It's recommended that you call the university to which you want to apply before you add the Extra choice, to check whether there is space on the course and to discuss your suitability. To apply for the new course, you need to add the details to your application.

Your chosen university will consider your application, and, if this is unsuccessful, you can add another Extra choice as long as it's before July. If you have not heard back from the university within 21 days, you can add another Extra choice (again, before July).

Once you have received an offer through Extra, you'll need to either accept or decline it. Ensure that you respond by the date displayed on your homepage, or your offer will be automatically declined.

Don't worry if you don't receive the offer you'd hoped for in UCAS Extra – you can still participate in Clearing.

What to do if things go wrong during the exams

Occasionally, students will underperform in an examination through no fault of their own. This could be through distressing family circumstances (a serious illness of a family member, for example), illness in the run-up to the exam (or during the exam), or unforeseen circumstances such as late arrival to the exam due to problems with public transport. In all cases, you should inform the universities that this has happened to you immediately after the examination. You should, if possible, get your referee to give the details to the universities and provide documentary evidence, such as a letter from your GP.

What to do on results day

You can collect your results from your school or college, or you can arrange to receive them via email or post. It's a good idea to go into school or college to receive them in person, so that you can get support and advice from teachers and careers advisers about your options if you need it.

UCAS receives your exam results directly and will update UCAS Hub with the outcome of your university applications on results day. The system will be busy, so you might need to be patient to find out whether you've been successful.

You'll need to have the following things ready to ensure that you can do everything you might need to on results day:

- UCAS Hub login details;
- UCAS ID number;
- UCAS Clearing number, if you go into Clearing;
- details of your offers;
- the UCAS and Clearing numbers of your chosen universities;
- a working phone and computer, so you can communicate by phone or email.

When you do get your results, one of four things will happen:

1. You receive confirmation of your place from the university you selected as your firm choice, and accept it.
2. You have not met the offer from your firm choice but you will receive confirmation from the university you selected as your insurance choice and accept it.
3. You have met and exceeded the offer made by your firm choice and decide to try to swap courses by going through Clearing (see below).
4. You have not met the requirements of any offers and need to go through Clearing.

If you have achieved the grades that meet the offer made by the university you selected as either your firm choice or insurance choice and are happy with this offer, then congratulations! You do not need to do anything. However, if you want to decline your firm place and make use of UCAS Clearing or have not met any offers and need to use Clearing, then read on.

What to do if you exceeded the grades that you expected

If you have met and exceeded the conditional requirements of your firm choice and it has accepted you – therefore converting the conditional offer into an unconditional one – you could potentially swap your place for one on another course that you prefer by using the 'decline my place' button in the application. The phrase 'met and exceeded' means that if you needed BBB you would have achieved ABB or better. It doesn't necessarily mean that you just got more UCAS points. For example, if you needed BBB and achieved A*BC, then you would have accumulated more UCAS points with A*BC than you would have if you had only achieved BBB. However, you would have still failed to meet one of your grade requirements. In cases like this, your eligibility will depend on whether your offer was based on UCAS points or grades.

If you decide to pursue a different course, you have to go through UCAS Clearing. Since more than 50,000 students get a course through Clearing, it is highly recommended that you find the course of your preference as soon as possible, as this is a first come, first served system.

Use the Clearing search tool to find all the available courses. Once you have found an alternative course, you will need to phone the university yourself. When you call the university, you will need to give them your UCAS personal ID number and explain straight away that you have exceeded the grades of your offers and are applying through Clearing.

Be prepared to answer questions about why you really want to study on that course. If they agree to accept you, and you in turn agree to accept them, this will happen during the phone call. Once you receive an offer, you can add it in your application so the college or university can officially accept you. At this stage, your status on UCAS Hub will change. Remember that if you do not find an alternative course that you want, or do not get accepted onto an alternative course, your original firm offer will still stand.

Make sure that you think carefully about the courses and universities, if you decide to go through Clearing. Just because a university has higher entry requirements or is considered to be more prestigious, it does not necessarily mean that you will enjoy the course more. Consider carefully why you selected your initial firm choice and check whether your reasons are still valid and you have the same interest and passion to study a new course.

What to do if you have no confirmed offers

If you are not holding any offers, there could be several explanations.

- You may have missed the required grades of both your firm and insurance offers.
- You may have achieved the right grades but not in the right subjects.
- The university or UCAS may not have received your results. The examination boards send the results automatically to UCAS, but if you sat an exam at a different centre, for example, then this may not have happened.
- The examination system that you sat does not automatically send the results to UCAS – for instance, if you sat overseas qualifications.

In the cases of achieving the right grades but not in the right subjects, contact your firm choice university to discuss this with it. Universities may revise their offer and admit you if they still have places, or if you missed the grade by only a few marks, they may ask you to try for a remark. Exam boards change the marks in only a few cases, though, and they can go down or up, so don't place all your hopes on this. If you still do not receive an offer from your firm choice university and have not received an offer from your insurance choice university, then call your insurance choice university. If, by the end of this process, you still have no offers, you will need to enter UCAS Clearing.

UCAS Clearing

Clearing is the name given to the system in which all remaining course vacancies are advertised on the UCAS website and in national newspapers. In Clearing, you contact the universities directly that have publicised course vacancies and give them your grades and UCAS ID number. If you think that you might need to use the Clearing system, it is best to be well prepared because the vacancies are filled very quickly. Clearing is typically open from July to October.

Alongside their search tool, which includes over 30,000 course options, UCAS also offers Clearing Matches, a tool that 'matches' candidates to a list of courses in UCAS Hub. If you find yourself in Clearing, it is advisable to check the 'See matches' button; if you find a course you like, select the 'I'm interested' button. If the university or college still has available places, they will contact you to discuss further and possibly make you an offer.

Advice for Clearing

- Make sure that you have your UCAS ID number and a copy of your UCAS application ready for results day.
- Remain proactive! Use the Clearing Matches tool to speed up the process of finding another place.
- You need to have access to a phone that you can use exclusively, as you may need to make a lot of calls over the course of results day.
- You also need to have access to the internet in order to access the directory of courses available through Clearing on the UCAS website. This is particularly useful as the website also has the university contact numbers that you will need to call.
- Think about the option of studying on courses that might not be identical to the one that you originally applied for, but are related.
- Be ready for an impromptu telephone interview. The admissions staff may ask why you want to study on the course, and you will need to have a little bit more tact than just saying 'because I didn't get into the course I really wanted to'. Instead, you could say something like 'Even though I didn't get into my firm or insurance choices I did apply/intend to apply/visit during the open day/ know that the course has a good student satisfaction rating in the *Guardian* and so on.'

If you decide to retake your A levels

If you have not achieved the grades that you needed for your chosen universities, and you do not want to take the available Clearing places, you could consider retaking one or more A levels. In the days when most examination boards offered January sittings, retaking might have meant studying for one term to boost the grade. The period from January to September could then be used to earn money, gain more work experience or travel the world. But, apart from international A levels, A level exams are now only available in June, and so retaking will involve studying for another year, so you need to be sure that your university aspirations are genuine enough to give you the motivation to add this extra year to your studies. As the A level system is now fully reformed, barring the last Phase Three legacy-subject examinations, you will need to retake the entire two-year qualification again and therefore plan to be able to do this in just a single year – you do not want a repeat of the examination if you are underprepared.

Speak to your teachers about the implications of retaking your exams. Some independent sixth-form colleges provide specialist advice and teaching for students. Interviews to discuss this are free and carry no obligation to enrol on a course, so it is worth taking the time to talk to their staff before you embark on A level retakes. Many further education colleges also offer retake courses, and some schools will allow students to return to resit subjects, either as external examination candidates or by repeating a year.

If you decide to reapply

Universities are usually happy to consider students who are reapplying, either because they did not get the required grades first time around, or because they did not receive any offers of places. It is worth contacting the university to check whether this is the case. Some will have policies on grade requirements for retake candidates, while others might ask for evidence of any extenuating circumstances that may have affected the previous application.

> **TIP!**
>
> If there were extenuating circumstances that affected your application, include a brief mention of this in the personal statement ('I was disappointed not to have achieved the required grades, because my studies were affected by illness, but this has made me even more determined to become an engineer') but leave the details to the referee.

If you are retaking, you can use the extra term or extra year to add weight to your application, for example by gaining more work experience, taking up a new subject, enrolling in evening classes that are relevant to your application and furthering your reading.

> **Fact**: Chocolate is poisonous to both cats and dogs. Surprisingly, it is the most effective type of mouse bait – mice don't really like cheese that much at all!

10 | Counting sheep
Financing your course

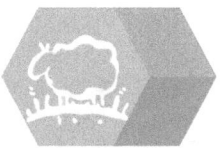

Whether undertaking an undergraduate or postgraduate course, the cost of studying is considerable. This has been exacerbated in recent years by rises in living costs and increases in university tuition fees. The UK Parliament's House of Commons Library released student loan statistics that revealed that, on average, students graduating in 2024 had a debt of £53,000.

NB, these figures are based on an average of all students, rather than focusing on veterinary students. As well as veterinary medicine courses being longer in duration, veterinary students have additional course-related expenses, such as travel expenses, placement fees, appropriate clothing, equipment and books. While many students might make the most of their holidays to work and earn additional money, veterinary students will have to spend most of their time on EMR/EMS placements in order to meet the prescribed experience required for their training.

On the whole, the cost of studying will fluctuate depending on:

- **Geographical location**: living in London will be more expensive than living in other cities in the UK.
- **Area of permanent residence**: there are differences in fees payable and the financial support available depending on your nationality.
- **Family support**: contributions from family members may significantly help reduce the costs accrued.
- **Availability of scholarships**: some universities provide financial support for students meeting particular criteria, such as academic excellence.
- **Part-time work**: this is difficult to manage while studying any course, but especially veterinary medicine; yet working while studying could help to reduce the overall burden of debt.

When considering levels of student debt, it is easy to become disheartened and think that university study is not for you. What all students must remember is that tuition fees do not have to be paid up front; in fact, most students receive student loans to cover this cost. In addition, the loans do not start to be paid back until you are earning over a certain amount. The full details of this will be discussed later in the chapter.

Regardless of how much debt you incur, or how you fund your way through university, hopefully the figures discussed below will help you to realise that undertaking a course such as veterinary medicine should only be done after seriously considering the overall cost and carefully examining your ability to be fully committed to your study for the full five years.

To find out what the fees are and what funding is available for veterinary medicine courses, you should explore each of the universities' websites and talk to their financial departments, because fees and funding procedures vary from university to university.

Fees

UK students

As the government of each of the UK home nations sets the fees that universities can charge, the tuition fees for undergraduate courses will depend on where you live and where you intend to study. In England, only universities with a Teaching Excellence Framework (TEF) award and an access and participation plan (APP) from the Office for Students (OfS) are permitted to charge the maximum tuition fee. However, the TEF's impact on tuition fees is specific to England: it does not affect fee caps in Scotland, Wales or Northern Ireland.

The maximum tuition fee for the 2025/26 academic year was increased to £9,535. Prior to that, the fee cap had been frozen at £9,250 since the 2017/18 academic year. In the autumn of 2025, the UK government announced that, from 2026/27, university tuition fees in England are set to increase every year in line with inflation. The Welsh authorities have confirmed that they will implement the same tuition fee increase as the UK government for the 2026/27 academic year, with the tuition fee cap for 2027/28 to be confirmed at a later date. At the time of writing (February 2026), Scotland and Northern Ireland are yet to confirm any plans to increase tuition fees for 2026/27 and beyond, so it is worth keeping an eye out in the news and on your regional student finance website for developments.

There are a number of variations between the systems in England, Scotland, Wales and Northern Ireland, which can result in significant differences between the fees that are ultimately paid by students. For reference, the current situation regarding tuition fees is as follows.

- Students from England will be required to pay maximum fees of £9,790 for 2026/27, rising to £10,050 for 2027/28.
- Students from Wales will be required to pay maximum fees of £9,790 for 2026/27, with increases in subsequent academic years yet to be confirmed.

- Students from Scotland who study at Scottish universities are not required to pay tuition fees. However, Scottish students who choose to study in other UK nations are required to pay the tuition fees set by that country.
- Students living in Northern Ireland paid up to £4,855 to attend university in Northern Ireland (2025/26). Northern Irish students who study elsewhere in the UK pay the tuition fees of that country.

International students

EU students are charged the same fees as charged to non-EU international students, which are significantly higher than those charged to UK students and are determined by each university. The RVC, for example, charges international students £50,360 per year from 2026 (which is subject to annual increases) and the University of Edinburgh's fees are £41,700 per academic year for overseas students who start their course in the 2026/2027 academic year. While there is some variation in cost between universities, these fees are broadly representative of the whole of the UK.

Some students from the EU may be eligible for some support in terms of student loans from the UK government, but this is dependent on a number of factors, so it is best to check personal eligibility. Students from the Republic of Ireland are exempt from paying higher fees and are eligible for home fee status.

Living expenses

Your living expenses include the cost of your accommodation, food, clothes, travel and equipment, leisure and social activities – plus possible extras like field trips and study visits, if these aren't covered by the tuition fees. See also Table 4 (overleaf) for details of expected expenditure on equipment for students applying to veterinary science courses.

Check university and college websites for information about possible living costs. Some are better than others and give breakdowns under various headings such as accommodation, food and daily travel. Others go even further and give typical weekly, monthly or annual spends.

If you're living away from home, accommodation will make up the largest proportion of your living costs. There is likely to be a range of accommodation options – from a standard room in university halls through to privately rented accommodation – with a range of price points. You'll probably be surprised when you do some research to find that the cheapest and most expensive towns are not as you might have expected; the cost of accommodation often depends on how much of it is available in a particular area.

Table 4 Typical costs for additional equipment required by veterinary students

Item	Typical Cost (2024/25)	Notes
Lab coat, waterproof trousers, boots and PPE	£50–£70	Usually purchased at the start of Year 1
Dissection kit, gloves, safety glasses, calculator	£40–£60	Often lasts the duration of the course
Basic stethoscope	£13–£25	Required from early clinical years
Yard or steel-toe boots	£30–£40	Essential for animal handling
Theatre shoes and clothing (final year)	£25–£30	One-off purchase
EMS placements (travel and accommodation)	£2,000–£2,500 total	May be higher if placements are distant
Average living costs outside London	£1,100 per month (around £13,500 per year)	Includes rent, bills, food and transport
Average living costs in London	£1,400 per month (around £17,000 per year)	Maintenance loans may not fully cover costs

When choosing accommodation, it is essential to consider its location and factor in the cost of travel to your university or college. It is also important to find out what's included in the accommodation costs (such as utilities, personal property insurance and Wi-Fi) and whether it is possible to pay for accommodation during term time only.

Funding

How do you fund your time in higher education? Don't ignore this question and leave it until the last minute! You will need to think carefully about how to budget for several years' costs – and you need to know what help you might get from:

- the government;
- your family or partner;
- paid part-time work;
- other sources, such as bursaries and scholarships.

This chapter gives a brief overview of a complicated funding situation, which can vary according to where you come from and where you plan to study. For more details about the different types of funding available and how to apply for them, check your regional student finance website:

- www.gov.uk/contact-student-finance-england
- www.studentfinancewales.co.uk
- www.saas.gov.uk
- www.studentfinanceni.co.uk.

Tuition fee loans

For UK students, tuition fees can be covered by taking out a tuition fee loan, which will be paid directly to your university or college at the start of each year of your course. You are effectively given a loan by the government that you repay through your income tax after you finish your course but only once your earnings reach a certain threshold. For 2026/27, these income thresholds stand at:

- £25,000 per year for students from England (Plan 5);
- £29,385 a year for students from Wales (Plan 2);
- £33,795 for students from Scotland (who go to university outside of Scotland) (Plan 4);
- £26,900 for students from Northern Ireland (Plan 1).

(All figures apply to students starting their course after 1 August 2023).

You only have to start student loan repayments once your earnings exceed the relevant threshold. In addition, any outstanding balance on your loan will be cancelled after a certain period of time if you have not already cleared it in full. The length of time depends on the rules at the time you took out the loan. For students in England who started their studies in September 2023, the repayment period was extended to 40 years (from 30 years), so it is recommended that students in other regions keep a close eye on any developments with respect to the length of the loan repayment period. At the time of writing, the loan repayment term is 30 years for students from Wales and Scotland, and 25 years for students from Northern Ireland.

Loan repayments are set at 9% of anything you earn over the annual income threshold.

The interest rate charged on student loans depends on what repayment plan you are on, but for students in England on Plan 5 it is currently 3.2%.

Maintenance loans

In addition to a tuition fee loan, all students can apply for a maintenance or living cost loan, which is repayable in the same way. All students are entitled to a maintenance loan; however, the amount you can borrow will be dependent on your household income – in other words, it is means tested. 'Household income' refers to your family's gross annual income (their income before tax). With the exception of loans available to Scottish students, the amount you can claim also varies depending on your living situation, with the maximum loan being available to students living away from home in London.

Each regional student finance website includes a finance calculator tool that will give an estimate of the finance you would be eligible for based on your family income and other factors, and it is well worth looking at this before planning your budget.

The government has announced that, from the 2026/27 academic year, maintenance loans for students from England will increase in line with inflation. Maintenance loans for Welsh students are also increasing; however, details of any additional support for students from Scotland and Northern Ireland for the 2026/27 academic year are yet to be confirmed. For reference, a summary of current maintenance support arrangements is given below.

England (2026/27)
The maximum annual maintenance loan in England:

- £9,118 for those living in the family home;
- £10,830 for those living away from home (£14,135 in London).

Wales (2026/27)
In Wales, students can get a combination of a maintenance grant, which they do not have to pay back, and a maintenance loan. Although the grants are means tested, most students should get a grant of at least £1,020.

The maximum amounts for maintenance loans and grants in Wales:

- £10,685 for those living in the family home;
- £12,590 for those living away from home (£15,720 in London).

Scotland (2025/26)
In Scotland, students can get a mix of maintenance loans and non-repayable bursaries (grants) to cover living expenses. These are as follows (all figures per year):

- Household income up to £20,999: £2,000 bursary and £9,400 loan;
- Household income £21,000–£23,999: £1,125 bursary and £9,400 loan;
- Household income £24,000–£33,999: £500 bursary and £9,400 loan;
- Household income £34,000 and above: no bursary and £8,400 loan.

Unlike the rest of the UK, household income for Scottish students is measured on the income bands listed above rather than exact household income.

The loan includes a Special Support Loan of £2,400, which is available to all full-time students. Unlike the maintenance loan and bursary, this is not means tested but it is repayable.

Northern Ireland (2025/26)

The maximum annual maintenance loan in Northern Ireland:

- £6,300 for those living in the family home;
- £8,132 for those living away from home (£11,391 in London).

In addition, you may be eligible for a non-repayable maintenance grant if your household income is below £41,065 and it is paid to you. This is paid alongside any maintenance loan you qualify for and is up to £3,475.

Scholarships and bursaries

In addition to government loans and grants, there are a number of non-repayable scholarships and bursaries available to veterinary students. These are offered both by universities and by external organisations that recognise the high costs of studying veterinary medicine and the importance of supporting new entrants to the profession.

Most universities offer hardship funds, access bursaries and academic scholarships. For example, the University of Nottingham provides a Veterinary Medicine Scholarship worth up to £7,500–£9,000 over the duration of the course for students from lower-income households, while the Royal Veterinary College (RVC) and the University of Liverpool offer bursaries to help with the extra costs of EMS placements and essential equipment.

Several external bodies and veterinary companies also provide awards:

- **VetPartners Bursary** – up to £1,500 per year for undergraduate veterinary students, awarded to those showing commitment, motivation and resilience.
- **RCVS Knowledge EMS Bursaries** – to help cover travel and accommodation costs during placements.
- **Vets4Pets and CVS Group Scholarships** – smaller awards (typically £500–£1,000) recognising academic excellence, research involvement or widening participation.
- **BVA Masters Bursary** – occasional support for undergraduate or early-career research projects.
- **RCVS Mind Matters and Diversity & Inclusion Funds** – small grants for projects promoting student wellbeing or equal access to the profession.

When applying, check each veterinary school's Fees & Funding webpage and note any deadlines or eligibility criteria. It's also worth searching sites such as www.thescholarshiphub.org.uk and the RCVS or BVA websites for updated lists of veterinary-specific support. Many awards are competitive, so apply early and ensure you meet the stated conditions, for instance, maintaining academic progress or continuing your studies in veterinary medicine.

Keeping costs down: hints and tips

Studying veterinary medicine is a major financial commitment, but there are plenty of ways to make your money go further. With a bit of organisation and planning, you can keep costs manageable while still enjoying student life.

- **Hold off on buying equipment or textbooks too early:** wait until you receive your official kit list and course guidance from your university. Many veterinary schools and student societies arrange bulk-buy discounts, and second-hand sales at the start of term are an excellent way to pick up items cheaply from older students.
- **Take advantage of student discounts:** apply for a TOTUM card, 16–25 Railcard or Young Person's Coachcard to save on everyday travel. Universities often have partnerships with local transport providers that offer reduced bus or train fares for regular travel to placements.
- **Apply for student finance early:** it can take several weeks for loans and bursaries to be processed, so make sure you apply well before the deadline. Having your funding confirmed in advance will make the start of term much smoother.
- **Budget by term or month:** create a realistic budget that includes rent, food, bills and placement costs. Apps such as Monzo, Cleo or Emma can help you track spending and set limits automatically, making it easier to stay on top of your finances.
- **Plan ahead for placements:** Extramural studies (EMS) placements are unpaid, and travel or accommodation costs can add up quickly. Check whether your university offers placement bursaries or whether you're eligible for support through schemes such as the RCVS Knowledge EMS Bursary.
- **Look for flexible part-time work:** while the course is demanding, some students successfully balance occasional weekend or evening work – for example, at local animal shelters, veterinary practices or pet shops. This not only provides extra income but also develops transferable skills and animal-handling experience.
- **Make Easter and summer count:** once you've completed your first lambing or farm placement, you may be able to earn £350–£400 per week doing seasonal agricultural work. It's challenging but rewarding, offering valuable experience and a welcome boost to your savings.
- **Share and swap resources:** many students share accommodation, lift-share to placements or rotate textbooks and lab equipment. Joining your university's veterinary society is a great way to connect with other students, exchange tips and find opportunities to save money.

10| Financing Your Course

Even with careful planning, studying veterinary medicine represents a significant financial investment. Before applying, it's sensible to understand what costs to expect – not only tuition fees and living expenses, but also the specialist equipment and placement costs unique to the course. The following section outlines some of the typical additional expenses veterinary students can anticipate and how these can vary depending on the university and location.

Alongside tuition fees, students should budget for living costs, course-specific equipment and placement expenses. Veterinary degrees are longer and more practical than most, so costs are often higher than in other subjects.

Average student living costs in the UK are now around £1,100–£1,250 per month, or roughly £13,500–£15,000 per year, depending on location and lifestyle. In London and parts of the South East, this can rise to £1,400 or more per month. Accommodation is likely to be your biggest expense, but other costs such as food, transport and study materials quickly add up.

Veterinary students also face additional expenses for protective clothing, clinical equipment and extensive travel for extramural studies (EMS) placements (see Table 4). Some of these costs can be reduced through bursaries, university hardship funds or EMS-specific support schemes.

Make use of your university's online budgeting tools to estimate termly spending, and plan ahead for placement periods when part-time work may be difficult. Buying second-hand textbooks, sharing accommodation and applying for early EMS bursaries can make a noticeable difference to your budget over time.

> **Case study**
>
> Bex is a third-year Veterinary Medicine student at the University of Surrey. Surrey was her first-choice university, so she was delighted to accept the offer to study there, which she secured by obtaining A*AA in chemistry, biology and geography at A level.
>
> 'My time at Surrey has been great so far; however, as with any vet course, there have been tough times! I am in my clinical years now, which I am finding very interesting. We are putting our Year 1 anatomy and Year 2 pathology knowledge into practice, learning how to problem-solve cases and treat them. At Surrey, we have been very hands-on from the start. In Years 1 and 2, we had animal-handling practicals and were in the anatomy labs a lot. This year, we have been learning how to do clinical skills, such as placing IV catheters, doing dentals, rasping horses' teeth – the list goes on!

'A specific area of interest of mine is equine veterinary. I have always loved horses, and when I first came to university, I even joined the polo team. My EMS placements have reinforced my passion for equine veterinary; for me, the placements are the most rewarding part of vet school. It is a chance to see everything that you have been learning in practice, and it aids your understanding of diseases and treatment protocols. I also find it incredibly interesting seeing how vets communicate with clients, especially in difficult cases. It is really the only place where you will learn this, and I think it is a great way to understand how to interact with different people in different circumstances.

'I think that the most challenging part of the degree is maintaining a good work–life balance. Sometimes the workload can feel overwhelming, but it is important to take time for yourself. It is very easy to get stressed about how much work there is to do: group projects, lecture notes, keeping on top of revision and so on. I overcome this by writing a short list each day of what needs to get done. Once I have gotten through the list, I can rest and do whatever I like for the rest of the day. I think that this is the best way to overcome having a never-ending list of things to do, which can easily make you feel overwhelmed and as if you are drowning in deadlines!

'My biggest tip for aspiring vets is to be organised. It is important to know what each university wants from you. I also found that doing a broad range of work experience really pushed me through my A levels, as it was a constant reminder of why I wanted to do well, and what my life could look like in the future. It gives you so much to talk about in interviews as well. Even if you aren't asked about work experience, it always looks good to pull from your previous experience to back your answers up.'

Fact: A puppy is born blind, deaf and toothless.

11 | Snakes and ladders
Career paths

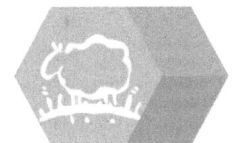

While training as a vet requires significant time, effort and financial investment, it also leads to a highly respected professional qualification and a wide range of rewarding career options. The majority of graduates initially enter clinical practice, but many later branch out into research, education, public health, government work and roles in industry or conservation.

According to the Royal College of Veterinary Surgeons (RCVS) Workforce Model 2023, around 80% of registered veterinary surgeons in the UK were working in clinical practice, with the remainder employed across academia, government agencies, charities and industry. The RCVS forecasts that this proportion will rise slightly, to around 83% by 2035, reflecting continued demand for veterinary professionals in companion animal, farm animal and equine sectors.

The RCVS has also reported growing interest among younger vets in non-traditional career paths, including wildlife medicine, global health, epidemiology and roles linked to sustainability and policy. This chapter explores these options in more detail, helping you understand where a veterinary degree can take you and how your career might evolve over time.

Veterinary Graduate Development Programme (VetGDP)

Graduation marks the start of your professional journey rather than the end of your training. Newly qualified vets in the UK now complete the RCVS Veterinary Graduate Development Programme (VetGDP), which replaced the former Professional Development Phase (PDP).

The VetGDP is designed to help graduates make a smooth and supported transition into professional practice. During this period, you'll work under the guidance of an RCVS-approved VetGDP Adviser, who will help you develop confidence and competence across a broad range of clinical and professional skills. These include areas such as animal handling, clinical reasoning, communication, teamwork and ethical decision-making.

You'll record your progress against the RCVS Day One and Year One Competences, reflecting on your experiences and identifying areas for further development. Completion of the VetGDP confirms that you are ready to work independently and continue building your skills throughout your career.

Beyond this initial phase, all registered veterinary surgeons are required to engage in Continuing Professional Development (CPD), a process of ongoing learning through courses, workshops, conferences and professional networking. This ensures that vets stay up to date with scientific advances, new techniques and best practice in animal health and welfare.

Once you've completed the VetGDP, you'll be well placed to explore the diverse range of veterinary career paths described in the rest of this chapter.

Career opportunities

Most veterinary graduates begin their careers in clinical practice, but one of the most appealing aspects of the profession is its diversity. A veterinary degree opens doors to a wide range of roles, both within traditional practice and far beyond it, and many vets change direction several times during their careers.

In the early years, new graduates typically enter companion animal, mixed, equine or farm animal practice, often within large multi-vet or corporate practices. There has been a steady trend towards small animal and companion animal medicine, reflecting the growth of pet ownership and the demand for advanced diagnostics and surgery. However, opportunities remain strong in farm animal practice, especially in herd health, welfare auditing and food production, and in equine practice, which continues to expand as part of the UK's leisure and sports industries.

Within practice, vets can also choose to specialise in particular clinical areas such as orthopaedics, dermatology, cardiology, neurology, anaesthesia or diagnostic imaging. Many go on to complete postgraduate qualifications through the RCVS Certificate and Diploma programmes or through postgraduate training schemes such as internships, residencies and European or American specialist board examinations.

Beyond practice, veterinary graduates are employed across a growing range of non-clinical roles. These include working for:

- government and public health agencies, for example, the Animal and Plant Health Agency (APHA), the Food Standards Agency (FSA) or Defra, focusing on disease control, biosecurity and food safety;

- universities and research institutions, contributing to biomedical research, teaching and advancing animal and human health through the One Health approach;
- pharmaceutical, biotech and nutrition industries, developing vaccines, diagnostics and therapeutics;
- charities and NGOs, promoting animal welfare and veterinary access in the UK and internationally;
- global health and conservation organisations, addressing zoonotic diseases, wildlife health and sustainability challenges.

Whether in a clinical, academic, industrial or policy role, vets play a crucial part in safeguarding both animal and human wellbeing. This flexibility means that a veterinary degree is not only a route to practice, but also a gateway to a wide range of rewarding and influential careers.

Postgraduate courses

Veterinary education doesn't stop at graduation. As a profession, it places strong emphasis on lifelong learning and Continuing Professional Development (CPD). All practising vets in the UK are required by the RCVS to complete a minimum number of CPD hours each year, but many also choose to pursue formal postgraduate qualifications to deepen their expertise or explore new areas of interest.

Postgraduate study is available in a wide range of formats, from part-time online courses to full-time master's or doctoral research degrees. These programmes allow vets and related professionals to build specialist knowledge in fields such as animal behaviour, infectious disease, public health, education or wildlife and conservation medicine. For example:

- University of Stirling offers an MSc in Aquatic Veterinary Studies for those interested in fish health and aquaculture.
- Newcastle University and the University of Edinburgh offer MSc programmes in Animal Behaviour and Welfare.
- University of Liverpool runs postgraduate certificates and diplomas in Veterinary Business Management and Veterinary Physiotherapy.

Many universities also offer research-based degrees (MRes, MPhil or PhD) that allow graduates to investigate topics ranging from zoonotic diseases to comparative neurobiology, immunology or One Health approaches.

Some vets undertake postgraduate qualifications accredited by the RCVS or European and American specialist boards (such as the European College of Veterinary Surgeons or the American College of Veterinary Pathologists). These are often completed as part of an internship or residency and lead to specialist registration within a particular discipline.

You do not need a postgraduate qualification to work as a vet, and most graduates enter practice directly after completing the Veterinary Graduate Development Programme (VetGDP). However, further study can be an excellent way to specialise, change direction or move into academia or research. It's usually best to gain a few years of professional experience first, so that you can make an informed decision about which area of veterinary medicine interests you most.

Veterinary variety: types of vet

The veterinary profession continues to evolve rapidly. There are now more practising vets in the UK than ever before, reflecting both the expansion of veterinary schools and a growing demand for animal care. However, the sector also faces ongoing challenges, from the rising cost of living for clients to workforce shortages and increased competition between independent and corporate practices.

As you progress through your degree, you'll begin to discover which aspects of veterinary medicine most appeal to you. Some students are drawn to the fast pace of small animal practice, while others prefer the variety of mixed practice, the technical demands of equine medicine or the population level problem solving of farm animal health and welfare.

It's usually recommended that new graduates begin their careers in general clinical practice, where they can develop a broad range of skills before specialising later on. Working with a mix of animal types early in your career helps build clinical confidence, improve communication with clients and deepen your understanding of the wider role vets play in animal welfare and public health.

From there, you can choose to focus your career in a particular species group or specialism, or even transition into a completely different area such as research, policy or education. The following sections outline the main types of veterinary practice and what each typically involves.

Small animal vet

Small animal practice remains the most common career path for veterinary graduates in the UK. According to the RCVS Workforce Model 2023, around 60% of practising vets now work mainly or entirely with companion animals such as dogs, cats, rabbits and other household pets – a steady increase over the past decade that reflects the UK's growing pet population and advances in veterinary healthcare.

As a small animal vet, you'll be responsible for providing preventative care, diagnostics and treatment for pets at local practices, animal hospitals or referral centres. Your work may include routine health checks, vaccinations, neutering and dental procedures, as well as emergency and surgical cases. You'll also play a key role in advising owners on nutrition, welfare and long-term health management.

The emotional side of the role can be challenging, particularly when it involves discussing quality of life or making end-of-life decisions with owners. However, it is also one of the most rewarding areas of veterinary medicine, offering the chance to build lasting relationships with clients and see the positive difference your work makes to the animals in your care.

Mixed practice vet

Mixed practice vets work with more than one type of animal – most commonly a combination of small animals, farm animals and horses. This type of practice is most often found in rural areas, where communities depend on veterinary services for both livestock and pets. The exact mix of work can vary widely from one practice to another, and even from one day to the next.

A typical day in mixed practice might involve vaccinating dogs in the morning, examining a horse for lameness after lunch and responding to a late-night calving emergency on a local farm. The variety makes this one of the most unpredictable but also the most rewarding areas of the profession.

Mixed practice allows new graduates to gain broad experience before deciding whether to specialise. It also helps develop a wide range of transferable skills, from clinical decision-making and communication to business management and adaptability, that can be valuable in any later career path.

The workload can be demanding, especially when out-of-hours duties are required, but many vets enjoy the close relationships they form with clients and the opportunity to work across species. As veterinary medicine becomes increasingly specialised, mixed practice continues to offer something unique: a career defined by variety, versatility and community impact.

Farm animal vet

Farm animal (or production animal) vets focus on the health, welfare and productivity of livestock such as cattle, sheep, pigs and goats. Rather than treating individual animals, their work usually centres on managing the health of the herd or flock as a whole.

Day-to-day responsibilities include diagnosing and treating disease, carrying out fertility checks, advising on nutrition and biosecurity and supporting farmers with herd health planning. A major part of the role involves preventative medicine, helping to reduce disease outbreaks and improve animal welfare through vaccination programmes, hygiene protocols and early intervention.

Farm animal vets play an essential role in maintaining the UK's food supply chain and protecting public health through disease control, food safety and traceability. They work closely with farmers, agricultural advisers and government agencies to ensure that livestock production is both ethical and sustainable.

This area of practice can be physically demanding, involving long hours and work in all weather conditions, but it is also highly rewarding. Many vets value the opportunity to form strong professional relationships with farming communities and to make a measurable difference to animal health and welfare on a large scale.

Equine vet

Equine vets specialise in the care and treatment of horses, ponies and donkeys. This area of practice combines aspects of sports medicine, surgery, internal medicine and preventative health, often with a strong focus on performance and welfare.

Equine vets typically work either in first-opinion practice, visiting yards, stables and riding schools to deliver routine healthcare, vaccinations, dentistry and lameness checks, or in referral hospitals, where they manage complex surgical or medical cases. Increasingly, the field also includes sports medicine, focusing on biomechanics, rehabilitation and injury prevention in competition horses.

Because horses differ from other animals in both anatomy and pharmacology, equine practice demands specialist knowledge and a confident, practical approach. Many equine vets begin in mixed or general practice before undertaking postgraduate training, such as an internship, residency or RCVS Certificate in Advanced Veterinary Practice (CertAVP) with an equine focus.

Equine practice can be physically demanding and often involves working irregular hours, but it is also highly rewarding. Vets in this field enjoy close partnerships with owners, trainers and riders, and play a vital role in promoting the health, welfare and performance of one of the UK's most iconic animals.

Exotic animal vet

Exotic animal vets specialise in the care of species other than traditional companion animals such as dogs and cats. The term 'exotics' covers a wide range of species, from reptiles, amphibians and birds to small mammals such as ferrets, guinea pigs and chinchillas. Some vets also work with zoo, aquarium or wildlife species, often in partnership with conservation organisations or academic institutions.

Because of the diversity of anatomy, physiology and husbandry across these species, exotic practice requires a strong grounding in general veterinary medicine as well as additional specialist training. Most vets begin in small animal practice before pursuing postgraduate certificates, residencies or diplomas in zoological or exotic animal medicine, often through the RCVS or the European College of Zoological Medicine.

The growing popularity of exotic pets in the UK has created increasing demand for vets with the skills to treat them. Veterinary schools are responding by expanding training in this area; for example, the Royal (Dick) School of Veterinary Studies in Edinburgh has established a dedicated Exotics and Wildlife Service, providing both clinical care and student training.

Exotic animal work can be technically challenging but hugely rewarding. It offers opportunities to combine clinical medicine, husbandry advice and conservation, while helping to promote better welfare for species that are often poorly understood by their owners.

Avian vet

Avian vets specialise in the care and treatment of birds – a group that includes everything from parrots, budgerigars and backyard poultry to raptors and zoo species. Because birds have unique anatomy, physiology and nutritional needs, avian practice requires a specialist skill set and a detailed understanding of each species' behaviour and husbandry.

Work in avian medicine can be incredibly varied. You might spend one day in private practice advising owners of pet birds, the next working at a sanctuary or wildlife rehabilitation centre and another supporting zoo or conservation projects. The variety of species and settings ensures that no two days are ever the same.

Most avian vets begin their careers in small animal or mixed practice before pursuing specialist training. Postgraduate qualifications such as the RCVS Certificate in Advanced Veterinary Practice (CertAVP) with an avian focus, or board certification through the European College of Zoological Medicine (Avian), are typical routes into the field.

As with other specialist areas, it's usually advisable to gain a few years of general clinical experience after graduation before undertaking avian or exotic qualifications. This helps you build strong diagnostic, surgical and communication skills that will serve as the foundation for your specialist training.

Other types of vet

The areas listed above (small animal, large animal, equine, mixed and exotic) are the most common career paths for newly qualified vets. However, these are far from the only options available. As you gain clinical experience, you can choose to specialise further in one or more areas of veterinary medicine, surgery or science.

Specialisation allows vets to develop advanced expertise, often through postgraduate qualifications such as the RCVS Certificate in Advanced Veterinary Practice (CertAVP), or through residency programmes leading to board certification with the European or American Colleges of Veterinary Specialists. Some vets also move into teaching, research or policy roles linked to their area of specialisation.

Below are examples of specialist areas currently recognised or commonly pursued in the UK:

Clinical and surgical specialisms
- anaesthesia and analgesia;
- dentistry (including equine dentistry);
- dermatology;
- diagnostic imaging (small or large animal);
- emergency and critical care;
- internal medicine (small animal, equine or farm animal focus);
- neurology;
- oncology (medical, surgical or radiation);
- ophthalmology;
- orthopaedics;
- soft-tissue and reconstructive surgery;
- sports medicine and rehabilitation.

Species-specific and production animal medicine
- cattle health and production (general, dairy or mastitis);
- pig medicine;
- poultry medicine and production;
- sheep health and reproduction;
- camelid health and production;
- equine reproduction and theriogenology;
- fish and aquatic animal medicine;
- feline medicine.

Population health, pathology and research
- epidemiology;
- pathology (anatomical, clinical, microbiological or zoological);
- pharmacology and toxicology;
- public health and food safety;
- parasitology.

Welfare, behaviour and conservation
- animal welfare, ethics and law;
- behavioural medicine;
- nutrition and clinical nutrition;
- wildlife and zoo medicine (mammal, avian, reptile or population health focus).

These specialisms reflect the breadth of modern veterinary science, extending well beyond traditional clinical practice. As technology and research continue to advance, new areas of expertise, such as veterinary data science, telemedicine and One Health collaboration, are also emerging, creating even more diverse opportunities for the next generation of vets.

The veterinary practice

There are many different types of veterinary practice, each offering a distinct working environment and caseload. The majority of practices in the UK are companion animal or mixed practices, though some focus solely on large animal or equine work. A smaller number specialise in areas such as referrals, exotics or emergency and critical care.

Practice sizes also vary widely. Many are small, independent surgeries with just two or three vets, while others are large, multi-vet hospitals or part of national corporate groups that operate multiple branches. Increasingly, new graduates may also encounter mobile clinics, telemedicine services and collaborative practices that share equipment and expertise across regions.

Whatever the setting, all practices share the same goal – to provide the best possible care for their patients and clients. Each practice has its own culture and rhythm: some are fast-paced and highly specialised, while others maintain a more relaxed community focus. As you explore potential career paths, you will begin to understand which type of environment best suits your working style and professional ambitions.

The structure of a general practice

In a general veterinary practice, the team works together to provide all types of care, from consultations and medical treatments to surgical procedures and preventative health. While each practice is unique, most follow a broadly similar structure, with defined roles that support both the animals and their owners.

Veterinary surgeons are at the core of the practice, diagnosing illness, performing surgery and prescribing treatments. Some vets also work towards additional qualifications accredited by the Royal College of Veterinary Surgeons (RCVS) while in practice, allowing them to specialise in areas such as surgery, internal medicine or diagnostic imaging.

New graduates often start as assistant vets (sometimes called associates or employed veterinary surgeons). In some independent practices, they may later progress to become partners, taking on part-ownership and business responsibilities. However, many practices are now part of larger corporate groups, where progression may instead lead to senior clinical roles such as clinical director or lead vet.

Practice managers play an increasingly important role in overseeing the day-to-day running of the business, from staffing and budgeting to compliance and client communication. In smaller practices, this role may be combined with that of the senior vet, but in larger ones it's usually a dedicated management position.

Registered Veterinary Nurses (RVNs) are essential members of the clinical team. They provide skilled nursing care, assist in anaesthesia and surgery, carry out laboratory work and help to educate clients about animal welfare and preventative care. Their role has expanded significantly in recent years, with greater autonomy and defined professional responsibilities under RCVS registration.

Receptionists and client-care assistants are the first point of contact for pet owners. They play a vital role in creating a welcoming, reassuring atmosphere and managing the flow of appointments and emergencies. Good communication from front-of-house staff helps maintain trust between clients and the clinical team.

Behind the scenes, many practices also employ animal care assistants, student veterinary nurses, laboratory technicians and administrative staff to ensure everything runs smoothly. Together, these individuals form a close-knit team, united by a shared goal – to deliver the best possible care to animals and their owners.

Veterinary practice as a small business

Veterinary practices are small businesses that rely on the income they generate from consultations, treatments and procedures. Unlike the NHS, veterinary care in the UK is not publicly funded, so each practice must cover its running costs, including staff salaries, rent, medical supplies, insurance and the upkeep of facilities and equipment, from the fees charged to clients. Any profit is reinvested into the practice to maintain standards and update technology.

Many vets, especially those early in their careers, are surprised by how much time and consideration goes into the financial side of practice. Even though the primary motivation for most vets is to care for animals, they also have a responsibility to keep the business sustainable so that they can continue to provide that care.

Vets often face difficult decisions when treating animals whose owners struggle to afford the necessary treatment. These situations can be emotionally challenging, as vets must balance animal welfare, client expectations and financial realities. Many practices try to support clients by offering staged payments, recommending pet insurance or referring them to charitable or low-cost clinics, such as those run by the PDSA, RSPCA or Blue Cross.

Understanding the business aspects of veterinary medicine, including how pricing, insurance and financial management work, is an important part of being a successful and compassionate professional. Whether you work in an independent clinic or a larger corporate group, being aware of both the clinical and commercial sides of practice will help you deliver better care for your patients and clients alike.

> **Did you know?**
>
> - Around 70% of UK veterinary practices are now owned by corporate groups such as IVC Evidensia, CVS, Linnaeus and Medivet. These companies manage multiple branches, allowing vets to focus more on clinical work while central teams handle marketing, HR and finance. Independent practices still exist, however, and often pride themselves on a close community feel.
> - Pet insurance is becoming increasingly common, with over 60% of dogs and 40% of cats in the UK now insured. Insurance can make advanced treatment options, such as orthopaedic surgery or MRI scans, accessible to more owners, but also shapes client expectations about the level of care available.
> - Many practices are exploring new business models, such as membership plans for routine care, mobile and telemedicine services and charitable partnerships that provide low-cost treatments. These developments are helping to make veterinary care more sustainable and more accessible for pet owners.

Accreditation

All veterinary practices and degree programmes in the UK must meet strict professional and regulatory standards to ensure the quality of animal care and veterinary education.

RCVS-accredited practice

The RCVS Practice Standards Scheme (PSS) is a voluntary accreditation system launched by the Royal College of Veterinary Surgeons (RCVS) in 2005. It sets out quality standards for veterinary practices across the UK, covering clinical governance, staff training, facilities, hygiene and client communication.

More than two-thirds of UK practices now hold RCVS accreditation, which demonstrates a commitment to continuous improvement and to delivering the highest standard of veterinary care. Practices can be accredited in one or more categories, such as small animal, equine, farm animal, emergency service clinic or hospital.

Working in an RCVS-accredited practice means you are part of a team that prioritises clinical excellence, animal welfare and ongoing professional development. You can read more about the scheme at www.rcvs.org.uk/pss.

BEVA-approved AI (artificial insemination) practices

The British Equine Veterinary Association (BEVA) maintains a register of veterinary surgeons and practices that perform equine artificial insemination (AI) and follow BEVA's Code of Practice. These standards ensure that AI procedures are carried out safely, ethically and in line with breeding regulations.

AVMA-accredited course

The American Veterinary Medical Association (AVMA) is the accrediting body for veterinary degrees in the United States and Canada. Graduates from AVMA-accredited programmes are eligible to sit the North American Veterinary Licensing Examination (NAVLE), which is required to practise in North America.

Several UK veterinary schools, including the Royal Veterinary College, the University of Glasgow and the University of Edinburgh, hold AVMA accreditation, meaning their graduates can work in North America without completing additional degree equivalence assessments.

EAEVE

The European Association of Establishments for Veterinary Education (EAEVE) evaluates veterinary schools across Europe to ensure their programmes meet agreed educational and professional standards. Many UK and European veterinary schools are either EAEVE-approved or hold RCVS-EAEVE joint accreditation, allowing greater international mobility for graduates.

For UK applicants, this system helps guarantee that your veterinary education meets the same rigorous professional benchmarks recognised across Europe and beyond.

Government and military service

Many vets work in the public sector, helping to protect animal health, public health and the safety of the food supply. These roles are vital for monitoring and controlling disease outbreaks, ensuring animal welfare during transport and slaughter and supporting sustainable farming practices.

In the UK, government-employed vets work across a number of departments and agencies, including:

- Defra (Department for Environment, Food and Rural Affairs) employs vets to monitor animal health and welfare, control notifiable diseases and manage disease-surveillance programmes.
- APHA (Animal and Plant Health Agency) formed in 2014 following the merger of the AHVLA and parts of the Food and Environment Research Agency (FERA). APHA vets work in the field and in laboratories to investigate disease outbreaks, carry out testing, enforce animal health regulations and provide advice to farmers and veterinary practices.
- Food Standards Agency (FSA) employs Official Veterinarians (OVs) who oversee meat hygiene, food safety and animal welfare in abattoirs.
- Veterinary Medicines Directorate (VMD) regulates the use, manufacture and licensing of veterinary medicines in the UK.
- UK Health Security Agency (UKHSA) and public health teams work with vets on issues that involve zoonotic (animal-to-human) diseases under the One Health framework.

Government vets play a crucial role in responding to outbreaks such as avian influenza or bluetongue, enforcing import and export regulations for live animals and animal products and advising ministers on animal welfare and biosecurity policy.

A career in the public sector can be extremely rewarding, combining veterinary expertise with policy, research and national-level impact. The Veterinary Public Health Association (VPHA) provides useful information about these roles and offers mentoring and training for those interested in this path.

Vets can also serve in the Royal Army Veterinary Corps (RAVC), where they care for service dogs and horses, contribute to public health and biosecurity and may undertake fieldwork or research. Officers typically join as Army Captains on a Short Service Commission (around four years), with opportunities to extend or transfer to a permanent commission. The role combines veterinary expertise with leadership, welfare and adventure, and offers fully funded postgraduate training and international deployment experience.

Veterinary teaching and research

Veterinary teaching and research are central to advancing our understanding of animal health, welfare and disease. Researchers in this field help improve the wellbeing of both companion and food-producing animals, while also protecting public health and contributing to breakthroughs that benefit human medicine through the One Health approach.

Research in veterinary science spans a wide range of topics, including infectious and zoonotic diseases, reproduction, cancer biology, genetics, neurology, nutrition and antimicrobial resistance. It also increasingly includes areas such as animal behaviour, climate change and biodiversity and veterinary education.

Most veterinary research in the UK takes place within the veterinary schools, in government laboratories and in research institutes and industry. The main funding bodies include the Biotechnology and Biological Sciences Research Council (BBSRC), Defra and UK Research and Innovation (UKRI).

A veterinary qualification offers many routes into research and academia. Some graduates remain in university settings, combining clinical teaching, research and specialist referral work. Others move into full-time research positions in universities, pharmaceutical companies or organisations such as the Animal and Plant Health Agency (APHA), Veterinary Medicines Directorate (VMD) or public health and biomedical research institutes.

Opportunities also exist to pursue further postgraduate study, such as MSc, MRes or PhD programmes, often focusing on specialist topics like epidemiology, neuroscience, immunology or comparative pathology. Many veterinary scientists work at the interface between human and veterinary medicine, making discoveries that improve healthcare for both animals and people.

Veterinary schools also host teaching hospitals and specialist referral centres, where cutting-edge clinical research is integrated into patient care. For example, advances in areas such as equine colic surgery, orthopaedic repair and neurological rehabilitation have stemmed from close collaboration between general practitioners and academic specialists.

A career in veterinary research and education is ideal for those who enjoy scientific discovery, problem solving and mentoring others, and who want to contribute to long-term improvements in animal and human health.

Charity and welfare organisations

Many vets choose to work for animal welfare charities, such as the RSPCA, PDSA, Blue Cross, Dogs Trust and Battersea Cats and Dogs Home. These organisations provide low-cost treatment, welfare inspections and rehoming services. Vets in this sector often balance clinical work with community education, policy advocacy or welfare investigations. It's a challenging but deeply rewarding field for those motivated by animal welfare and social impact.

Non-clinical veterinary careers

While most graduates begin their careers in clinical practice, an increasing number discover rewarding roles outside traditional veterinary settings. These career paths still make full use of your veterinary training, but they focus less on day-to-day clinical work and more on science, policy, communication or management. For some vets, this direction offers a better work–life balance, more predictable hours or the chance to specialise in the wider impact of animal health on society.

Here are some of the most common non-clinical roles taken up by veterinary graduates:

Public health and government roles

Vets play a crucial part in protecting human and animal populations at a national and international level. Roles include:

- government veterinary services (APHA, Defra, FSA) working on disease surveillance, animal welfare, food safety and biosecurity;
- public health roles monitoring zoonotic diseases and ensuring standards in the food supply chain;
- international work with bodies such as the World Organisation for Animal Health (WOAH) or the World Health Organization (WHO), focusing on One Health issues.

These roles suit graduates interested in policy, population health and disease prevention.

Pharmaceutical and biomedical industries

Many vets work within the pharmaceutical, biotechnology and diagnostics sectors. Roles include:

- research and development of new medicines, vaccines and diagnostic tests;
- pharmacovigilance, monitoring medicine safety after release;
- technical advisory positions, supporting vets and practices in using new products.

These roles often involve research, scientific communication and working closely with industry partners.

Laboratory diagnostics and pathology

Some vets move into roles focused on laboratory analysis, disease investigation and interpreting diagnostic tests. Careers include:

- veterinary pathologists working in specialist labs;

- diagnostic roles in private laboratories, universities or government agencies;
- research support in areas such as infectious disease or genetics.

This route suits students who enjoy problem solving and investigative work.

Animal welfare, charities and non-profits

Vets are central to many animal welfare organisations, including the RSPCA, Battersea, Dogs Trust, Blue Cross and international charities. Work may involve:

- policy development and advocating for welfare standards;
- education and outreach programmes;
- fieldwork in areas such as population management, rescue and rehoming.

These roles can be highly fulfilling for those motivated by advocacy and community impact.

Education, science communication and consultancy

Vets contribute to public engagement, education and training through:

- teaching roles in universities or colleges;
- writing, broadcasting and content development (including advisory roles for media);
- consultancy in areas such as behaviour, nutrition, farming or biosecurity.

This path may appeal to graduates who enjoy communication, mentoring or outreach.

Why consider non-clinical careers?

Non-clinical roles offer:

- more predictable working hours compared to on-call clinical practice;
- the chance to influence animal health at a population rather than individual level;
- opportunities to specialise early in a niche area;
- the ability to combine veterinary expertise with other interests, such as research, policy or education.

Many vets move in and out of clinical and non-clinical roles throughout their careers, demonstrating the breadth and flexibility of the profession.

Veterinary salaries and career progression

When considering a career in veterinary medicine, it's useful to understand how salaries typically progress, but also important to remember that salary is only part of the picture. Pay varies widely depending on experience, area of practice (small animal, farm, equine, mixed, referral/specialist), location, employer (independent vs corporate), working hours and additional responsibilities (emergency work, business ownership, specialisms).

Typical salary ranges (UK, 2024-25)

- Newly qualified vets (one to three years' experience) usually earn base salaries in the region of £40,000–£45,000.
- Established general practice vets with several years of experience often earn £50,000–£65,000+ per year.
- Senior vets, clinical directors or practice owners, especially in larger or referral practices, may earn £70,000–£90,000 or more depending on the size and profit of the business.
- Specialist vets (with advanced qualifications, referral work or niche expertise) may command salaries of £80,000+, reflecting their high level of skill and responsibility.
- For example, a recent industry survey reported a mid-range median of £65,000 and a high-range median above £82,000 for senior roles in mid-2025.

What affects pay?

- **Practice type and size**: corporate groups may offer structured pay scales, while smaller independent practices might include profit sharing or partnership routes.
- **Species focus and specialism**: small animal work is often more common, but farm, equine, exotic or referral work may come with different pay scales and demands (including out-of-hours duties).
- **Location**: practices in London and the South East typically pay more to reflect higher living costs; rural or remote practices may offer incentives (housing, relocation) to attract vets.
- **Additional roles and responsibilities**: emergency cover, out-of-hours shifts, senior clinical roles, management or partnership often bring extra pay or profit share.
- **Career development**: vets who build their skills, gain additional qualifications (e.g. certificates, diplomas, specialist training) and take on leadership or referral roles generally see stronger salary growth.

How to use this information

- **Set realistic expectations**: if you're applying to vet school, know that your early-career salary will be modest compared to later stages – the big rewards often come with experience, specialism and responsibility.
- **Focus on progression**: think about how you will develop your career – what species you'd like to work with, whether you might specialise or whether you might aim for a leadership or referral role.
- **Consider work–life balance**: a higher salary often comes with more demands (e.g. emergency work, longer hours, larger responsibility). Consider what kind of lifestyle you want.
- **Ask good questions at interviews**: when applying for jobs, ask about salary progression, bonus or profit-share schemes, payment for out-of-hours, support for training and specialism.
- **Remember salary isn't everything**: job satisfaction, support, training opportunities, location, company culture and personal development are just as important – many vets say they stay in the job because of these, not just pay. In fact, only 42% of vets in a recent survey rated their pay and benefits as good or better.

Case study

Hannah is a small animal vet who studied at the University of Nottingham and has been working in a small animal practice ever since.

'I always knew I wanted a career that would combine science, problem solving and compassion, and veterinary medicine turned out to be the perfect mix. Since graduating from Nottingham, I've worked in a busy small animal practice in Norfolk, where no two days are ever the same.

'Some days are non-stop surgery lists, others are filled with consults and emergency cases. I really enjoy the investigative side of the job, trying to piece together what's going on when an animal can't tell you what's wrong. I've developed a real interest in internal medicine and imaging, and I'm currently studying for my postgraduate certificate in diagnostic imaging alongside full-time practice. Lifelong learning is a big part of being a vet – the more you learn, the more you realise how much there still is to know!

'The job can be emotionally demanding at times, especially when it comes to euthanasia or dealing with clients who are struggling with difficult decisions. But I've learnt that empathy and clear communication are just as important as clinical skills. Supporting an owner through a hard moment can be one of the most meaningful parts of the job.

'The biggest surprise for me has been how collaborative the profession is – from vet nurses to reception teams to referral specialists, you're never working in isolation. It really is a team effort.

'I'd tell anyone thinking about becoming a vet to go into it with your eyes open. It's challenging and sometimes exhausting, but it's also deeply rewarding. There's nothing quite like seeing an animal you've treated make a full recovery and walk back through the door a few weeks later wagging its tail. That moment always reminds me why I wanted to do this in the first place.'

Veterinary nurses

Veterinary nurses play a vital role in every practice, working alongside veterinary surgeons to deliver high-quality care for animals. Their responsibilities range from monitoring anaesthetics and assisting in surgery to performing diagnostic tests, administering treatments and supporting owners with advice on animal care and husbandry.

Many nurses also take on managerial or teaching roles, helping to train student nurses and new staff members and ensuring that clinical standards are maintained. Others move into research, universities, zoos, rehabilitation centres or animal welfare charities, reflecting the wide variety of career paths available.

Training routes

To become a registered veterinary nurse (RVN), you must complete an RCVS-approved qualification and register with the Royal College of Veterinary Surgeons. There are two main training routes:

- **Vocational route**: the Level 3 Diploma in Veterinary Nursing, studied full-time or part-time while working in an approved training practice. This route suits students who prefer hands-on, practical learning.
- **Higher-education route**: a Foundation or Bachelor's degree in Veterinary Nursing, studied at university. These degrees often include academic modules in animal science, behaviour or rehabilitation, alongside clinical placements.

Both routes lead to the same professional qualification and RCVS registration, though the degree pathway may open further opportunities in research, education or management later in your career.

Course length and placements

Most veterinary nursing courses take three years to complete, though some universities offer a four-year 'sandwich' degree that includes an integrated placement year in practice. All courses include a substantial clinical placement component, known as clinical training hours, which must be completed in an RCVS-approved training practice (TP).

Where to study

There are now more than 20 universities and colleges across the UK offering RCVS-accredited veterinary nursing degrees or diplomas. Examples include:

- Harper Adams University, offering degrees in small animal, equine and companion animal nursing;
- Hartpury University, with integrated placement years;
- Nottingham Trent University, which combines clinical and behavioural science;
- Middlesex University, which offers both direct-entry and Foundation-Year routes.

For the most up-to-date list of accredited veterinary nursing qualifications, visit the RCVS website: www.rcvs.org.uk/veterinary-nurses

Career progression

After qualification, veterinary nurses can develop further through clinical specialisms (such as anaesthesia, emergency and critical care or feline nursing), or move into practice management, teaching, research or welfare work. With experience, nurses may train as Advanced Veterinary Nurses (AVNs) through postgraduate study, or even become Practice Managers or Lecturers in veterinary education.

> **Did you know?**
>
> - The demand for qualified veterinary nurses has grown steadily across the UK, with many practices reporting staff shortages, meaning strong job security for new graduates.
> - In 2023, the RCVS reported that over 90% of newly registered veterinary nurses found employment within six months of qualifying.
> - Veterinary nurses are taking on increasingly advanced clinical responsibilities, such as leading nurse consultations, performing schedule 3 procedures (minor surgeries under veterinary supervision) and managing anaesthesia in complex cases.
> - Experienced RVNs can go on to gain postgraduate qualifications in areas like anaesthesia, emergency and critical care, behaviour, rehabilitation or feline nursing.
> - New routes such as Advanced Veterinary Nurse (AVN) status and clinical leadership roles are creating more opportunities for progression within the profession.

Women in the profession

The veterinary profession has changed dramatically over the past 40 years. Once a male-dominated field, it is now one of the most female-dominated professions in the UK.

According to UCAS End-of-Cycle data for 2024, around 78–80% of applicants to veterinary medicine were female (see Table 5), a trend that has remained consistent for several years. This pattern is reflected in the wider profession – the RCVS 2024 Workforce Report found that over 62% of practising UK vets are now women, and more than 80% of veterinary nursing professionals are female.

While women now make up the majority of new graduates and early-career practitioners, gender imbalances persist at senior levels. The Society of Practising Veterinary Surgeons (SPVS) reported in 2024 that the gender pay gap within UK veterinary practice remains around 19–21%, largely reflecting differences in seniority, ownership and working hours rather than starting salaries.

Encouragingly, both the British Veterinary Association (BVA) and RCVS are actively addressing these disparities through initiatives promoting leadership development, flexible working and mentorship schemes aimed at improving progression into senior clinical and managerial roles.

As the demographic shift continues, the profession is benefiting from a more diverse workforce, with increasing numbers of women in research, policy, academia and specialist practice as well as in clinical roles.

Table 5 UCAS 2024 end-of-cycle applicant statistics for Pre-clinical Veterinary Medicine: male and female applicants

	Applications	Accepted applicants
Men	2,280	290
Women	9,080	1,250
Total	11,360	1,540

Wellbeing in the veterinary profession

A career in veterinary medicine can be incredibly rewarding, but it is also recognised as one of the most emotionally and psychologically demanding professions. While many vets experience a strong sense of purpose and fulfilment, the profession also faces higher-than-average levels of stress, burnout and mental health challenges. It is important for aspiring vets to be aware of these realities, not to discourage you, but to help you enter the career with your eyes open and equipped with strategies for maintaining wellbeing.

Understanding the pressures

Several factors contribute to the demands of the job:

- **Emotional responsibility**: vets regularly deal with sick, injured or terminally ill animals, and must support owners during difficult decisions, including euthanasia.
- **High workload and long hours**: many practices are busy, with vets balancing clinical work, administration, EMS supervision and ongoing CPD requirements.
- **Client expectations**: with the rise of social media and online reviewing, vets can face pressure from clients who may expect immediate answers or feel distressed about treatment costs.
- **Financial considerations**: some new graduates feel tension between providing gold-standard care and clients' ability to pay, which can lead to moral stress.
- **Isolation**: in some environments, particularly rural or sole-charge positions, vets may feel professionally isolated.

These pressures do not affect everyone equally, but they are well recognised across the profession.

Support within the profession

The veterinary community has taken significant steps to improve wellbeing and foster supportive working environments. Examples include:

- **RCVS Mind Matters Initiative (MMI)**: provides resources, training, mental health awareness and campaigns aimed at reducing stigma and encouraging help-seeking.
- **Vetlife**: a confidential service offering emotional support, mental health assistance and financial help for vets, nurses, students and their families. Their 24/7 helpline is widely used across the profession.
- **Wellbeing policies within practices**: many practices now adopt structured rotas, protected CPD time, mentoring for new graduates and clearer expectations around work–life balance.
- **Graduate support schemes**: the RCVS Graduate Development Programme (GDP), introduced in 2021, ensures new vets are supervised, supported and given structured development rather than left to 'sink or swim'.

These systems are helping to shift the culture and provide better scaffolding for early-career vets.

Building resilience as a student and graduate

It is never too early to begin developing habits that support your wellbeing. Strategies include:

- **Seeking mentorship**: whether through university schemes, EMS hosts or supportive lecturers.
- **Developing healthy coping strategies**: exercise, hobbies, socialising and regular breaks are crucial to balance demanding workloads.
- **Setting realistic expectations**: no vet knows everything; recognising limits and asking for help is an essential professional skill.
- **Strengthening communication skills**: effective communication with clients can reduce misunderstandings and stress.
- **Prioritising rest**: fatigue significantly affects judgement, confidence and emotional resilience.
- **Using available support services early**: counselling, academic advisers and university wellbeing teams are there to help.

Students who engage with support services and develop balanced routines early tend to adjust better in clinical environments.

A career with meaning

Despite the challenges, many vets describe their work as deeply fulfilling. Helping animals, improving welfare, solving complex problems and supporting communities bring a sense of purpose that continues throughout a career.

Understanding the realities – the highs and the pressures – helps you enter the profession informed, prepared and resilient. You will not face the journey alone: support is embedded throughout the veterinary community, and developing healthy habits during your training will help you thrive in this demanding and rewarding career.

Summing up

Many students dream of becoming veterinary surgeons. For some, it will remain an aspiration, not because they lack potential, but because the path demands dedication, resilience and a realistic understanding of what the profession involves. However, for those who are motivated, compassionate and determined, there are genuine opportunities to succeed.

Competition is intense but not insurmountable. Early exploration through work experience, volunteering and talking to practising vets or vet nurses will help you understand the realities of the role – the long hours, the responsibility and the emotional challenges, but also the immense rewards.

The best preparation is curiosity, practical experience and a willingness to keep learning. A veterinary career offers not only variety, but also the chance to make a real difference to animals, people and the planet.

The demand for veterinary services and research expertise remains strong and continues to grow, driven by advances in animal welfare, food security and One Health initiatives linking animal, human and environmental health. The number of veterinary school places in the UK is influenced by both workforce demand and university funding and capacity, but the profession continues to attract a high level of interest from applicants each year.

For most, the appeal lies not in financial reward or lifestyle convenience, as veterinary work can involve long and unpredictable hours, but in the profound sense of purpose and variety that comes with the role. Increasingly, practices are supported by shared out-of-hours and emergency services, helping to improve work–life balance, but the profession still demands dedication and adaptability. For many vets, it remains more than a job – it's a vocation and a way of life.

The unique skills a vet requires

A vet is many things – a skilled clinician, problem solver, communicator and advocate for animal welfare. They must combine scientific knowledge with empathy, critical thinking and the ability to make difficult decisions. Vets know that the animals they treat are often a central part of their clients' lives, and they carry a deep responsibility for their health and wellbeing.

The role demands resilience, compassion and professionalism. At times, vets must make complex ethical judgements – balancing animal welfare, client expectations and practical realities. They also need strong business awareness and teamwork skills, as modern practice involves collaboration with nurses, receptionists, technicians and specialists.

It is a challenging career, but also an immensely rewarding one. If you have the curiosity, compassion and commitment to pursue it, veterinary medicine offers the opportunity to make a real difference every single day.

Fact: Horses can't vomit.

12 | Don't count your chickens before they've hatched

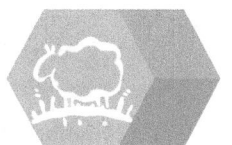

Further information

Don't fall into the trap of assuming you already know enough – there is always more to learn, and researching your options thoroughly will make you a far stronger applicant. Taking the time to understand the differences between courses, campuses and teaching styles will help you make an informed decision and give you confidence when speaking to admissions teams.

Reaching out to universities with thoughtful, specific questions is always worthwhile. Admissions tutors appreciate applicants who show genuine curiosity and have clearly researched the programme. A well-prepared question is remembered for the right reasons.

Below you will find the contact details for all UK veterinary schools, along with useful websites and organisations to support your research.

Veterinary schools in the UK

Aberystwyth
School of Veterinary Science
Penglais Campus
Penglais
Aberystwyth
Ceredigion SY23 3FL
Tel: 01970 623111
Email: vet-info@aber.ac.uk
Website: www.aber.ac.uk/en/vet-sci

Bristol
Bristol Veterinary School
Langford House
Langford
Bristol BS40 5DU
Tel (veterinary admissions): 0117 428 2744

Email: bvs-exec-admin-team@bristol.ac.uk (general enquiries); choosebristol-ug@bristol.ac.uk (admissions); vet-student-admin@bristol.ac.uk (veterinary queries)
Website: www.bristol.ac.uk/vetscience

Cambridge
Department of Veterinary Medicine
University of Cambridge
Madingley Road
Cambridge CB3 0ES
Tel: 01223 337701
Email: enquiries@vet.cam.ac.uk
Website: www.vet.cam.ac.uk

Edinburgh
Royal (Dick) School of Veterinary Studies
University of Edinburgh
Easter Bush Campus
Midlothian EH25 9RG
Tel: 0131 651 7305
Email: vetug@ed.ac.uk
Website: www.ed.ac.uk/vet

Glasgow
Admissions Office
School of Veterinary Medicine
College of Medical, Veterinary and Life Sciences
University of Glasgow
Garscube Campus
Bearsden Road
Glasgow G61 1QH
Tel: 0141 330 5706
Email: reception@vet.gla.ac.uk
Website: www.gla.ac.uk/schools/vet

Harper & Keele
Harper Adams University site
Newport
Shropshire TF10 8NB
Tel: 01952 815100
Keele University site
Staffordshire ST5 5BG
Tel: 01782 731844
Email: admissions@hkvets.ac.uk
Website: www.harperkeelevetschool.ac.uk

Lancashire
Admissions Office
School of Veterinary Medicine
University of Lancashire
Fylde Road
Ashton-on-Ribble
Preston PR1 2HE
Tel: 01772 892400
Website: www.lancashire.ac.uk/schools/veterinary-medicine

Liverpool
School of Veterinary Science
Leahurst Campus
Chester High Road
Neston
CH64 7TE
Tel: 0151 794 4797
Email: vetadmit@liverpool.ac.uk
Website: www.liv.ac.uk/veterinary-science

London
The Registry
Royal Veterinary College
University of London
Royal College Street
London NW1 0TU
Tel: 020 7468 5147
Email: admissions@rvc.ac.uk
Website: www.rvc.ac.uk

Nottingham
Admissions Team
School of Veterinary Medicine and Science
University of Nottingham
Sutton Bonington Campus
College Road
Sutton Bonington LE12 5RD
Tel: 0115 951 6116
Email: veterinary-enquiries@nottingham.ac.uk
Website: www.nottingham.ac.uk/vet

SRUC School of Veterinary Medicine
Scotland Rural College
Craibstone Estate
Aberdeen
AB21 9YA
United Kingdom.
Tel: 0800 269 453
Email: facultyofficeaberdeen@sruc.ac.uk, study@sruc.ac.uk
Website: www.sruc.ac.uk/veterinary-medicine

Surrey
School of Veterinary Medicine
Faculty of Health and Medical Sciences
Vet School Main Building (VSM)
University of Surrey
Daphne Jackson Road
Guildford
Surrey GU2 7AL
Tel: 01483 68 2222
Email: vetschool@surrey.ac.uk
Website: www.surrey.ac.uk/school-veterinary-medicine

Other contacts and sources of information

Useful organisations and professional bodies

Animal Welfare Foundation (AWF)
www.bva-awf.org.uk
Supports animal welfare education and research.

Blue Cross
www.bluecross.org.uk
UK charity providing animal hospitals, behavioural support and rehoming.

British Equine Veterinary Association (BEVA)
www.beva.org.uk
Professional association for equine veterinary surgeons.

British Small Animal Veterinary Association (BSAVA)
www.bsava.com
Professional body offering training, CPD and resources for vets and vet nurses.

British Cattle Veterinary Association (BCVA)
www.bcva.org.uk
Specialist association for farm animal veterinary professionals.

British Veterinary Association (BVA)
www.bva.co.uk
The national representative body for the veterinary profession.

Department for Environment, Food and Rural Affairs (Defra)
www.gov.uk/government/organisations/department-for-environment-food-and-rural-affairs
Animal health policy, notifiable diseases and biosecurity information.

PDSA (People's Dispensary for Sick Animals)
www.pdsa.org.uk

SPVS – Society of Practising Veterinary Surgeons
www.spvs.org.uk
Provides business, leadership and wellbeing support for vets.

VDS Training (Veterinary Defence Society)
www.vds-training.co.uk
Workshops and courses on communication, professionalism and wellbeing.

Vet Record (BVA journal)
https://bvajournals.onlinelibrary.wiley.com/journal/20425205

World Organisation for Animal Health (WOAH)
www.woah.org

Royal College of Veterinary Surgeons (RCVS)
Belgravia House
62–64 Horseferry Road
London SW1P 2AF
Tel: 020 7222 2001
Email: info@rcvs.org.uk
Website: www.rcvs.org.uk

Useful RCVS links:

- Find a Vet: www.findavet.org.uk
- Education and accreditation: www.rcvs.org.uk/education
- Overseas registration: www.rcvs.org.uk/registration

International veterinary schools

St George's University (Grenada)
University Centre
Grenada, West Indies
Tel (UK enquiries): 0800 169 9061
Email: sguenrolment@sgu.edu
Website: www.sgu.edu

University of Veterinary Medicine and Pharmacy in Košice (Slovakia)
Komenského 73
041 81 Košice
Slovakia
Tel: +421 915 984 004
Email: study@uvlf.sk
Website: www.uvlf.sk

Government and public sector bodies

DAERA – Department of Agriculture, Environment and Rural Affairs (Northern Ireland)
www.daera-ni.gov.uk

UK Government Student Finance
www.gov.uk/student-finance

Student resources and support

UCAS – Universities and Colleges Admissions Service
www.ucas.com

The Student Room
www.thestudentroom.co.uk

MRCVS Online Directory
www.mrcvs.co.uk

WikiVet
https://en.wikivet.net

Courses, virtual work experience and events

VetCam (University of Cambridge)
www.vet.cam.ac.uk/study/vet/vetcam
Tel: 01223 330811
Two-day residential 'Introduction to Veterinary Science' course.

Vetsim (Workshop Conferences)
www.workshop-uk.net/vetsim
Annual conference for aspiring veterinary students.

FutureLearn – Veterinary Online Courses
www.futurelearn.com/courses/vet-school-application-support
Virtual work experience widely recognised by vet schools.

RVC Veterinary Virtual Work Experience
www.rvc.ac.uk/study/undergraduate/vet-vwex

Publications

Getting into Oxford & Cambridge: 2027 Entry, Matthew Carmody, Trotman.
HEAP 2027: University Degree Course Offers, Brian Heap, Trotman.
How to Complete Your UCAS Application: 2027 Entry, Ryan Moran & UCAS, Trotman.

Glossary

Admissions tutor
The member of university staff responsible for assessing applications and making offers.

American Veterinary Medical Association (AVMA)
The professional body for veterinarians in the United States. It accredits some international veterinary degrees and provides professional guidance and resources.

Animal and Plant Health Agency (APHA)
The government agency (formerly AHVLA) working on behalf of Defra across Great Britain. APHA monitors animal health and welfare, conducts laboratory testing and manages disease control.

Animal husbandry
The care, breeding and management of livestock.

Bachelor of Veterinary Medicine/Veterinary Medicine Degrees
UK veterinary degrees have different titles depending on the university (BVetMed, BVMS, BVSc, VetMB). Cambridge awards a BA after three years and the VetMB after six.

Bovine spongiform encephalopathy (BSE)
A fatal neurological disease in cattle, often called 'mad cow disease'. The related human disease is variant Creutzfeldt–Jakob disease (vCJD).

Bovine tuberculosis (bTB)
A chronic infectious disease of cattle caused by *Mycobacterium bovis*. Wildlife, particularly badgers, can act as reservoirs of infection, contributing to ongoing debate around control measures.

British Equine Veterinary Association (BEVA)
The UK's leading professional body for equine veterinary surgeons, providing training, CPD and guidance.

Clinical years
The final years of the degree focused on hands-on practical training, rotations and clinical skills.

Continuing Professional Development (CPD)
Ongoing training required by the RCVS. Vets must complete at least 35 hours per year (or commit to this average over three years).

Department for Environment, Food & Rural Affairs (Defra)
The UK government department responsible for agriculture, environment, animal health and welfare, and food safety.

Department of Agriculture, Environment and Rural Affairs (DAERA)
The Northern Ireland government department responsible for agriculture and animal health (formerly DARDNI).

European Association of Establishments for Veterinary Education (EAEVE)
Organisation responsible for evaluating and accrediting veterinary degree programmes across Europe.

Extramural studies (EMS)
Work experience undertaken outside the vet school. As of the new RCVS framework (2023):

- Pre-clinical EMS: 12 weeks
- Clinical EMS: 26 weeks

Students must complete a minimum of 38 weeks of EMS.

Extramural rotations (EMR)
Structured placements undertaken outside the university, usually during clinical years, to develop applied clinical skills.

Foot-and-mouth disease (FMD)
A severe viral disease affecting cloven-hoofed animals such as cattle, pigs and sheep. Highly contagious but not a risk to human health.

Federation of Veterinarians of Europe (FVE)
A pan-European federation representing veterinary organisations across Europe.

Integrated course
A course structure that blends multiple scientific disciplines throughout the degree instead of teaching them separately.

International English Language Testing System (IELTS)
A standardised English-language proficiency test. UK vet schools typically require IELTS 7.0 overall with minimum scores in each component.

Intramural rotations (IMR)
Clinical training rotations that take place within the university's teaching hospital and associated facilities.

Master of Science (MSc)
A postgraduate degree that may be taught or research-based, typically completed in one to two years.

Methicillin-resistant *Staphylococcus aureus* (MRSA)
A strain of bacteria resistant to many antibiotics. Primarily associated with human healthcare settings but can infect animals.

Multiple-choice questions (MCQs)
A common assessment format used in many veterinary exams.

North American Veterinary Licensing Examination (NAVLE)
The licensing exam required to practise veterinary medicine in the United States and Canada.

Glossary

People's Dispensary for Sick Animals (PDSA)
A UK veterinary charity providing free or low-cost treatment and running pet hospitals.

Pharmacodynamics
How drugs affect the body.

Pharmacokinetics
How the body absorbs, distributes, metabolises and excretes drugs.

Pre-clinical years
The first two years of the veterinary degree, focusing on foundational science such as anatomy, physiology and pathology.

Professional Development Phase (PDP)
The structured experience and skills-recording phase undertaken immediately after graduation. Replaced by the RCVS Veterinary Graduate Development Programme (VetGDP) in 2021.

RCVS: Royal College of Veterinary Surgeons
The regulatory body for vets and vet nurses in the UK. It oversees professional conduct, accreditation of courses and registration.

Royal Society for the Prevention of Cruelty to Animals (RSPCA)
A leading animal welfare charity involved in rescue, campaigning and enforcement.

Royal Veterinary College (RVC)
The UK's oldest veterinary school and part of the University of London.

Therapeutics
The use of medications to treat or prevent disease.

UCAS
The centralised application service for UK university admissions. Applicants may choose four veterinary courses plus one non-veterinary choice.

Veterinary Medicines Directorate (VMD)
The UK government body responsible for regulating veterinary medicines and ensuring their safe and responsible use.

Veterinary Defence Society (VDS)
A mutual insurance company providing professional indemnity insurance and training for veterinary surgeons.

Fact: 'The quick brown fox jumps over a lazy dog' – it does this while using every letter of the alphabet.

Have you seen the Getting into University series?

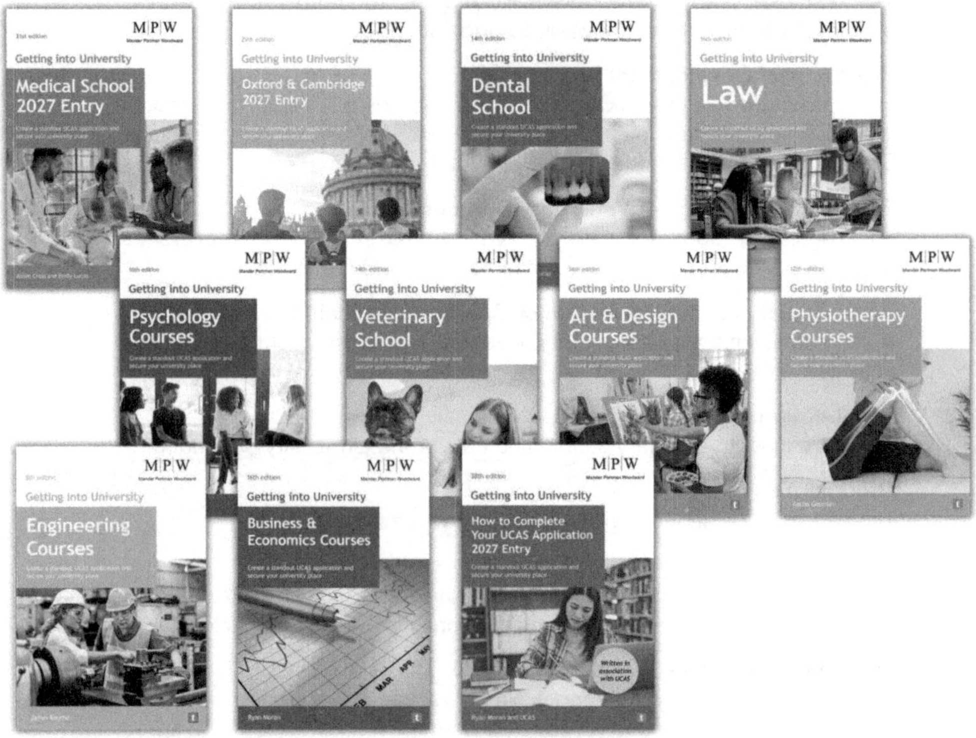

Get 30% off with code GET30

Our best-selling guides go beyond the official publications to give you expert, practical advice on how to successfully secure a place on the university course of your choice.

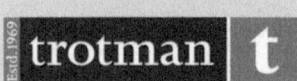

Order today from
www.trotman.co.uk/GettingInto